Play, Physical Activity Public Health

Are children playing less than they used to? Are rising obesity rates linked to a decline in children's time to play freely? These and other related questions have filled the pages of newspapers, magazines and scholarly journals for the past decade. Researchers and journalists have attributed these issues to societal changes around children's lives and leisure, the growth of structured and organised activities and increasing perceptions of risk in children's play. *Play, Physical Activity and Public Health* presents a discussion of the way modern notions of play are rendering children's leisure activities less free and less engaged in simply for fun.

Based on original qualitative research, and analysis of contemporary media from Canada and elsewhere, this book argues that the growing health concerns around childhood play entail a paradox: by advocating, promoting, discussing and re-directing children's play, a new form of children's leisure is emerging – one that is purpose-driven, instrumentalised for health and, ultimately, less free. We explore how play has become goal-oriented, a means to health ends, and how the management of pleasure in play as well as diverse risk discourses around play continue to limit and constrain possibilities for children and families to play and engage in leisure freely. Incorporating past critiques of this trend in play, we argue for research and practice to create new possibilities and ways of thinking about children's play, leisure, fun and childhood that are less constrained and managed and importantly less geared towards health goals.

This is a valuable resource for students of the sociology of sport, kinesiology, sports and health psychology, education, public health and childhood studies. It is also an important read for school teachers, public health practitioners, psychologists, physical education teachers, academics and parents interested in how children's leisure lives are being shaped by the growing and diverse discussions around play.

Stephanie A. Alexander is Post-doctoral Fellow at the Collège d'études mondiales in Paris, France in the Chair *Anthropology and Global Health*.

Her research involves critical examinations of interventions on children's play and physical activity to analyse how play may be reshaped when it is promoted for health purposes. Her current research examines questions about the globalisation of concepts such as 'active play' and of assumptions about childhood and health that underlie physical activity interventions.

Katherine L. Frohlich is Professor with the Département de médecine sociale et préventive within the École de Santé Publique at Université de Montréal (ESPUM), Canada as well as Research Associate with the Institut de Recherche en Santé Publique at Université de Montréal (IRSPUM). She is Director of the Masters Programme in Public Health at ESPUM. Her current research interests include social inequities in health-related practices, the sociology of smoking and the playability of urban spaces.

Caroline Fusco is Associate Professor in the Faculty of Kinesiology and Physical Education at the University of Toronto, Canada. She favours post-structuralist, feminist and cultural geography theories and her work is grounded in the pursuit of ethical relations, equity and social justice. Her current research interests centre on the cultural landscapes of play, youth and ecologies of urban recreation, intersectional studies of sport, sexuality and space, and she is most passionate about bringing a critical animal studies lens to the disciplines of kinesiology, recreation and sport.

Routledge Studies in Physical Education and Youth Sport
Series Editor: David Kirk
University of Strathclyde, UK

The *Routledge Studies in Physical Education and Youth Sport* series is a forum for the discussion of the latest and most important ideas and issues in physical education, sport and active leisure for young people across school, club and recreational settings. The series presents the work of the best well-established and emerging scholars from around the world, offering a truly international perspective on policy and practice. It aims to enhance our understanding of key challenges, to inform academic debate and to have a high impact on both policy and practice, and is thus an essential resource for all serious students of physical education and youth sport.

Also available in this series:

Examination Physical Education
Policy, Pedagogies and Possibilities
Trent D. Brown and Dawn Penney

Digital Technology in Physical Education
Global Perspectives
Edited by Jeroen Koekoek and Ivo van Hilvoorde

Redesigning Physical Education
An Equity Agenda in Which Every Child Matters
Edited by Hal A. Lawson

Play, Physical Activity and Public Health
The Reframing of Children's Leisure Lives
Stephanie A. Alexander, Katherine L. Frohlich and Caroline Fusco

For more information about this series, please visit: www.routledge.com/sport/series/RSPEYS

Play, Physical Activity and Public Health

The Reframing of Children's Leisure Lives

Stephanie A. Alexander,
Katherine L. Frohlich and
Caroline Fusco

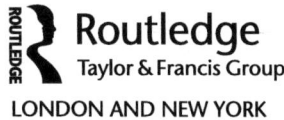
LONDON AND NEW YORK

First published 2019 by Routledge

2 Park Square, Milton Park, Abingdon, Oxfordshire OX14 4RN
52 Vanderbilt Avenue, New York, NY 10017

Routledge is an imprint of the Taylor & Francis Group, an informa business

First issued in paperback 2019

Copyright © 2019 Stephanie A. Alexander, Katherine L. Frohlich and Caroline Fusco

The right of Stephanie A. Alexander, Katherine L. Frohlich and Caroline Fusco to be identified as authors of this work has been asserted by them in accordance with sections 77 and 78 of the Copyright, Designs and Patents Act 1988.

All rights reserved. No part of this book may be reprinted or reproduced or utilised in any form or by any electronic, mechanical, or other means, now known or hereafter invented, including photocopying and recording, or in any information storage or retrieval system, without permission in writing from the publishers.

Notice:
Product or corporate names may be trademarks or registered trademarks, and are used only for identification and explanation without intent to infringe.

British Library Cataloguing-in-Publication Data
A catalogue record for this book is available from the British Library

Library of Congress Cataloging-in-Publication Data
A catalog record for this book has been requested

ISBN: 978-1-138-28972-7 (hbk)
ISBN: 978-0-367-89626-3 (pbk)

Typeset in Sabon
by Apex CoVantage, LLC

To my nieces, who all play better than I do. (SA)

To my son Oscar for all I learned from him and his love of unstructured play. (KF)

To my son Liam and beautiful dogs Finnegan and Seamus – their joyful play has sustained me over the last 14 years. (CF)

Contents

Acknowledgements   x

1   The play paradox   1
2   Playing as progress   26
3   Active play: when playing becomes a job   46
4   Playing is fun! (. . . or is it?)   76
5   Risk, play and free-range kids   98
6   Playing just makes me happy   129

Index   150

Acknowledgements

A conversation Kate had with her friend Sarah Watson many moons ago about play and children was the conception of this project. Kate wishes to thank Sarah for starting that conversation with her. And to Thomas Schlich for his constant constructive input on Kate's musings about this project.

Caroline thanks Kathleen Gallagher for her constant support and advice to "write about what you care about" and her two co-authors, who invited her on this initial journey just over 10 years ago, and who have demonstrated a playful collegiality throughout.

Stephanie wishes to thank Kate and Caroline for their mentorship, ideas and support over the past 10 years. Stephanie also wishes to thank her cohort of colleagues and friends who supported her, both with play and patience, over the course of this project. Last, she thanks her Montreal and Paris writing groups for their very helpful feedback on various iterations of this work.

We all would like to acknowledge the time that the children and families gave to us when data collection was being undertaken. We also would like to thank the Social Sciences and Humanities Research Council, SSHRC (Grant Number: 491116) for their funding of part of this work and for a SSHRC and an AXA-France post-doctoral fellowship (to SA). We also thank Routledge for their guidance in the process of publishing this book.

Chapter 1

The play paradox

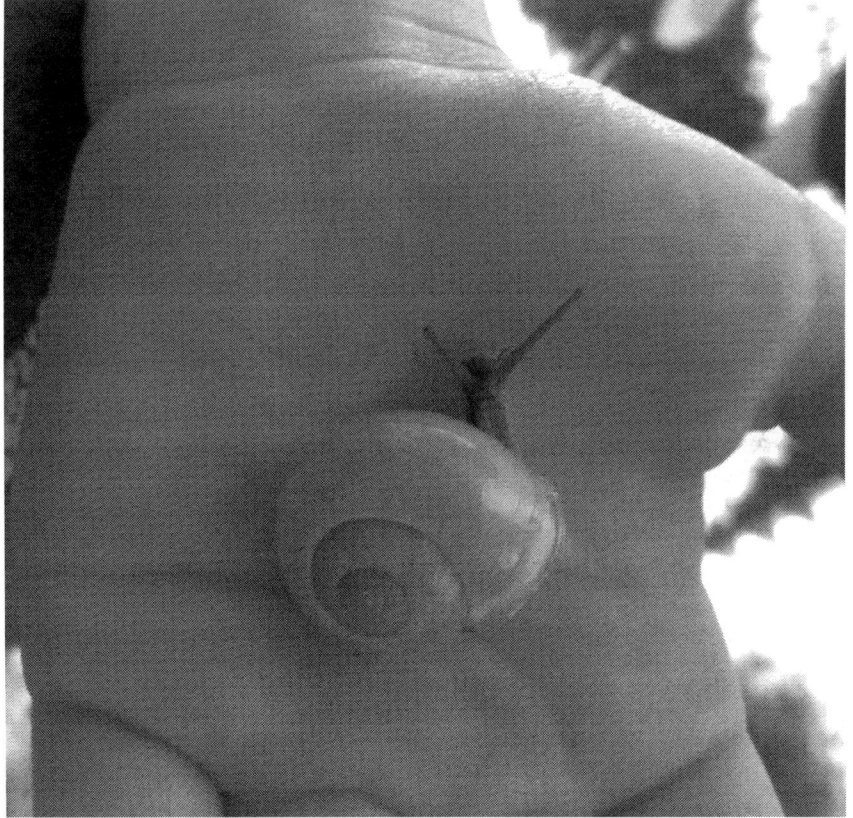

Figure 1.1 Alisha (8 years old) took a photo of Rapido, her pet snail.

Introduction

Are children playing less today than they used to? Are rising obesity rates among children in countries of the global north linked to the changing nature of children's play and the reduced time, space and freedom they have to play? Questions such as these have filled the pages of newspapers, magazines and scholarly journals for almost a decade. Concomitantly, around 10 years ago, play advocates, researchers and journalists also began expressing concerns about children's changing play culture attributing declines in *free* play to both societal changes and those regarding our perceptions of childhood. It was also at this time, in 2008, that one of the authors of this book (S. Alexander) began her PhD with one of her supervisors (K. Frohlich). Both of us became interested in these emerging discussions around children's play in Canada and specifically the emerging interest in children's leisure and play within Canadian public health.

In this book we discuss how ideas about childhood, health and play have begun to shift the nature of contemporary children's play activities. In the context of widespread calls for children's play to be protected and further promoted, we examine whether the engaged and organised promotion of children's play may in effect make children's play *less* free and *less* of an activity done "simply for fun". We argue that the growing physical health concerns around children, and the promotion of explicitly healthy play entails a paradox. By advocating, promoting and re-directing children's play towards activities that have a productive health end (i.e., physically active play) or that are predominantly safety-oriented, a new form of play seems to be emerging; one that is purpose-driven, risk-free, instrumentalised and, above all, *less* likely to be free. In this book we focus specifically on the development of the public health interest in play and trace the diverse events and circumstances that led up to the writing of the book. We outline the confluence of discussions, concerns and changes around childhood, children's health and their leisure activities, and the subsequent development within public health of a focus on children's play to promote physical activity.

In this first chapter, we introduce the "raison d'être" of the book: our curiosity and concern about the way playing was increasingly being conceptualised and then introduced into public health discourses. We briefly introduce some of the themes that fuelled our interest in the topic of children's play and outline the theoretical framing of our research, including the concepts and lenses through which we analysed the current situation of play. We also present the methodologies we drew on to concretely examine children's play. Finally, we provide an outline for each of the chapters of the book.

Where did our interest in play come from?

The year 2008 was a defining year for what would be our work on children's play within public health, and indeed, for Canadian discussions around children's play more generally. It was that year that one of the book's authors (S. Alexander) began her PhD with another of the authors (K. Frohlich) at the Université de Montréal's School of Public Health in Canada. While discussing research topics, both observed that the issues and concerns around children's "disappearing play" was becoming increasingly conspicuous and, indeed, hard to ignore. Whether it was the opinion pieces about declines in children's spaces to play written up in national newspapers or scientific magazines (e.g., Chouinard, 2006, *Le Devoir*; Wenner, 2009, *Scientific American Mind*), interviews about the consequences of "play deficit" for children on radio or television programmes (e.g., McDonald, 2009, *Quirks & Quarks*; Kennedy, 2009, *CBC Ideas*; Harper, 2009, *CTV*) or the publication of several books highlighting the critical importance of play for psychological (and overall) well-being of children (e.g., Brown, 2009; Elkind, 2007; Honoré, 2009), the topic of children's play, concern about its decline and an emphasis on the need to salvage it was omnipresent. This diverse body of knowledge was pointing to the emergence of a more general concern about the ways in which children play.

That same year, a Canadian non-profit organisation that evaluates and promotes children's physical activity (*Active Health Kids Canada*) published their fifth annual *Physical Activity Report Card for Children and Youth*, and for the first time included the concept of "active play" as an indicator for children's physical activity (we discuss this development further in Chapter 3). While previously relatively little had been discussed about the physical health benefits of children's playing – much more was written about the psychological and social benefits of play – new discussions within public health were beginning to address the physically active elements of specific kinds of playing. Bearing witness to the emerging interest in children's play from within our own discipline, we decided it was imperative to examine this more closely. Given that the interest in play was new within public health, we sought collaboration with the third author of this book, C. Fusco, an early-career researcher in *Kinesiology and Physical Education* (University of Toronto) at the time, to examine the introduction of children's play into public health from a broader perspective. Dr. Fusco was studying children's narratives about active school transport and the spaces of young people's physical activity (Fusco, Moola, Faulkner, Buliung, & Richichi, 2012; Fusco, 2007) and was interested in joining our examinations of play. We all entered the world of play by reading broadly on the historical transformations around play in the 18th, 19th, and 20th centuries and by examining play from multiple disciplinary perspectives. Our concern was to examine how the object of play came to be a significant component of children's physical activity promotion within the larger field of Canadian public health.

Since 2008 – a good 7 years before we began writing this book – the notion of play as a public health concept and indicator for physical activity has only continued to proliferate and circulate. In 2015, for instance, a new position statement (which will be discussed in Chapter 5) was developed and written up to address and confront the general societal tendency toward the avoidance of risky outdoor active play. In 2016, the Lawson Foundation funded 18 projects across Canada as part of an *Outdoor Play Strategy* to promote children's outdoor free play, active play and risky play. Children's play has thus become a central component of physical activity and public health agendas. The PhD research therefore followed this momentum developing around play within public health and physical activity organisations since 2008. The project examined both the dominant perspectives on play and juxtaposed these with children's own perspectives about their play preferences. To position the public health trends regarding play more broadly, this research also historically examined how contemporary ideas and concerns about play, health, physical activity and childhood developed in other fields (i.e., education, psychology, sociology of childhood) and how some of these were taken up by public health interventions to promote a form of physically active play.

The current book includes much of this work, but additionally draws on and includes new material and debates on childhood and play as these have continued to emerge in public health, physical education and popular discourses since 2014 when the PhD research was completed.

Children's play in transformation

Our historical lens on the transformation of play over the last century or so has been informed largely by a diverse group of historians and play theorists (e.g., Baker, 2001; Caillois, 1961; Chudacoff, 2007; Frost, 2010; Gutman & de Coninck-Smith, 2008; Huizinga, 1949; Read, 2011; Schwartzman, 1976; Stearns, 2005; Sutton-Smith, 1981, 1997). Their histories of play have specifically examined how societal shifts have affected children's lives and their play activities, and how this has altered the meanings attributed to playing. One of the most eminent 20th-century historians of play, Johan Huizinga, wrote the renowned book *Homo Ludens* (1949) which outlines his theory of play and its role in the development of western civilization. Huizinga's reflections on play were strongly influenced by societal changes in early 20th-century Europe, which included the expansion of industrialisation, the aftermath of the First World War and the growing wave of nationalism and fascism that would eventually lead to the Second World War (Anchor, 1978). While his general critique of modern civilisation makes itself heard in *Homo Ludens* (e.g., "we have seen great nations losing every shred of honour, all sense of humour, the very idea of decency and fair play" p. 205), the critique of modern life recorded in *Homo Ludens* focuses specifically on the declining role attributed to play in his contemporary society (i.e., early 20th century). What emerges as especially prominent in Huizinga's work is his observation that the play element, something he argues has always existed in society, was beginning to wane. He argues that already, as of the late 19th century, play in academic settings and schooling had begun to decline, and there was a growing tendency to "view play as something not quite respectful" (p. 192).

While Huizinga writes about the changes in play more generally, including adult play, contemporary historians writing about the 19th and 20th centuries have also observed changes, specifically with regard to children's play and its impact on psychological and social development. These more recent discussions centre on shifts from what many call unstructured and freer play in diverse play spaces, to forms of play that are increasingly structured, highly organised and adult-supervised. Play activities that were not explicitly fulfilling an aim (i.e., learning, development) began to be viewed as unproductive and were already being rejected in the early 20th century in favour of "good" productive play (Chudacoff, 2007; Frost, 2010; Read, 2011).

Play research has also been prominent in studies of children's schooling, sport and physical education. While these studies are too numerous to mention here, we acknowledge some of the scholars who have developed the wealth of literature on critical studies of physical education (Dowling, Fitzgerald, & Flintoff, 2012; Evans, Davis, & Wright, 2004; Evans, Rich, Davis, & Allwood, 2008; Whitehead, Telfer, & Lambert, 2014; Wright & Harwood, 2009) and those who have problematised children's participation in sport, recreation, play and physical activity (Dagkas & Armour, 2012; Dagkas & Burrows, 2016; Eichberg, 2017; Green & Smith, 2016;

Harvey & Light, 2013; Parker & Vinson, 2013; Wright & Macdonald, 2010). Historically, it has been organised sports activities that have been seen as more purposeful, productive and community oriented than play and as such, children, particularly middle-class children, were ushered towards sport, recreation and leisure activities, which do not necessarily include play experiences (Human Kinetics, 2013). While children have always engaged in play and leisure, and have played sports and games in various societies (Kamphorst & Roberts, 1989), in western industrialised nations, child and youth sport has become a billion-dollar industry (Gatz, Messner, & Ball-Rokeach, 2002). Child and youth sports were originally organised around the beliefs about what sport could provide for children – character development, teamwork and commitment (Holt, 2008; Gatz et al., 2002), and there is a wealth of literature on the rise of child and youth sports in the USA, Britain, Canada, Australia and New Zealand (Kremer, Trew, & Ogle, 1997). Specifically, children and youth were encouraged to engage in individual or team sports, and were less encouraged to simply engage in leisure play, take part in risky sports or become involved in counter-culture activities, although that trend is changing (Reinhart, 2014; Thorpe, 2012). Furthermore, as less space was made available for free play and leisure outdoors because urban planning began to design children out of street spaces (Moore, 1987), more children were harried into cars and driven to local arenas, playing fields, baseball diamonds and recreation centres (Thompson, 1999). With this, attention turned away from the provision of time and space for unstructured free play.

The success of child and youth sports in the latter half of the 20th century is undeniable, but now more than ever this path to play(ing) is being questioned. Children's sports have been riddled with concerns about the welfare of young people in those sports, the abuse of young athletes by coaches and highly competitive parents (Atkinson, 2009; Brackenridge, Pitchford, Russell, & Nutt, 2007; Lang & Harthill, 2015), the anti-social traits that can be learned through youth competitive sport (Atkinson, 2009) and, finally, the culture of risk-taking and injury that is perpetuated in youth sports, particularly masculine-identified sports (Kehler & Atkinson, 2010). Additionally, organised youth sport has succeeded in dividing children in terms of their sex/gender, social class, racialization and abilities (Azzarito & Macdonald, 2016; Messner, 2011). Although, play may (re)produce these divisions (Gagen, 2000), in and of itself, it is not organised along the same lines as competitive youth sports and recreation (Frost, 2010; Torkildsen, 2005), and in fact distinguishes itself from sports, leisure and recreation. However, Torkildsen (2005) argues that although play "has developed its own playwork career structure distinct from leisure and recreation", it is the cornerstone of children's leisure, recreation and free time (p. 6). Likewise, Cordes (2013) suggests that play is at the core of leisure (i.e., residual-time not work oriented) and recreation (i.e., activity that people engage in during their free time, that people enjoy, and that people recognise as having socially redeeming values), but that leisure and recreation appear to be more associated with community life, whereas play does not have to be.

Furthermore, while some child and youth sports are played outdoors and not in contained gyms (e.g., soccer, baseball, football), outdoor playing fields, like indoor gymnasiums, are highly regulated spaces in terms of rules, time and surveillance of risk, and these spaces rarely allow for children's spontaneity and agency in the way that free play does (IPA, 2016). Certainly, organised sports and recreation do not allow children and youth to "turn the world upside down" or allow space for them to "create uncertainty"; some of the fundamental characteristics of children's play (Lester & Russell, 2014).

All of these socio-cultural contexts and concerns around sports and recreation have in fact led to a drop in registrations for many traditional sports in Canada (Gruneau, 2010; Jeske Crane, 2014; Strashin, 2016), and this may be the reason why there has been such a refocusing on, and increasing promotion of, children's free play.

Our central argument

The public health interest in play has therefore unfolded against the backdrop of transformations in children's play, sport, leisure and recreation that occurred over the course of the 19th and 20th centuries, and it appears to be further informed by converging areas of contemporary research on children's physical health. First, current research suggesting that there are decreasing opportunities for children to play actively outdoors, and that this changing context for children's leisure activities may have consequences for children's physical health, is significant for public health. Second, the growing concerns about the increasing rates of childhood obesity appear to be driving public health efforts to find solutions to children's inactivity. Lastly, the trends showing that children are engaging in new forms of leisure, including screen and computer play, which are deemed risky, have further informed public health interventions on children's play. Play is therefore taken up and actively promoted within public health institutions, but in a particular form: as a physical activity that has as its principal aim the production of an optimal, healthy and safe childhood.

In this book we argue that while promoting the physical health of children is a critically important aim, the possible consequences of increasingly emphasising play as a health practice ought to be questioned. We ask how this physical health perspective applied to children's play may affect children's own experiences of playing. We explore the ways in which play is becoming a goal-oriented activity, a means to a specific end, deemed a necessity for children's optimal physical health and development. We demonstrate how institutions of public health are shaping what is considered the "correct" way to play and question how this is affecting the ways children engage in, and understand, their own play. When play becomes productive for health, or is made to fit a schedule – in short when play becomes efficient, compartmentalised and productive – the affective value that children attribute to play activities (i.e., the pleasure and spontaneity) may be transformed.

The interrelated transformations in children's play outlined previously introduce the various elements of the argument we make in this book and highlight how the diverse discourses on children's play have produced a glaring – and difficult to avoid – paradox. That is, while play is valued as a freely chosen and pleasurable activity for children, it is predominantly discussed and promoted for its beneficial *outcomes*, particularly with respect to children's health and development. We argue that this instrumentalisation of play specifically *for* physical health, and the overall focus on play as productive, runs the risk of reshaping children's play experiences, and children's social lives more generally. Drawing on sociologically and historically informed conceptions of play, we suggest that circumscribing play, and promoting it as an instrument for learning, socialising, improving cognitive abilities and for improving physical health, transforms play into an activity that is anything but free.

Furthermore, we consider how viewing play primarily through a productive health optic may also narrow the scope of what play can mean (i.e., relevant only for health and development) and thus also what can be included within its scope (i.e., play as active, healthy). This is a process Meyer and Schwartz (2000) call the "public healthification" (p. 1189) of the social, which they liken to the well-known concept of "healthism" (Crawford, 1980, 2006; Skrabanek, 1994). This "public healthification" of social practices is not new, as we will discuss in Chapter 4, however, its application to children's play is. Referring to some of the defining characteristics of play, Sydnor and Fagan (2012), draw on Huizinga's original conception of play as foundational for society and argue that play in this broad conception is "a limitless epistemology, ontology, method" for reconciling "our human need for story with the paradoxical, incomprehensible (plotless) nature of what it is to be human – and nonhuman" (2012, p. 79). They argue that "without play, the universe would be stagnant" (p. 78), and suggest that play thus has a creative role for society and cannot (should not?) be altogether tamed or ordered or specifically productive for anything at all. We consider, from a public health perspective, whether this role for play as "creative for society" is being done away with in the drive to promote forms of play for children that are productive and efficient in attaining health goals.

The popularity of the obesity epidemic discourse (Gard & Wright, 2005; Rail, 2012; Wright & Harwood, 2009) and the growing urgency to address global childhood obesity rates, has resulted in, among other initiatives, the development of yearly report cards in Canada outlining children's physical activity patterns as well as mediatised campaigns targeting children's sedentary leisure, all of which are further discussed in Chapter 3. As a sign of its global appeal, these report cards are now also being released by researchers and organisations in 38 countries, all of whom are similarly evaluating and promoting children's physical activity levels in their respective countries (Active Healthy Kids Global Alliance, 2017). This attention has jettisoned children's physical (in)activity and play to the forefront of the public health-driven campaigns to combat childhood obesity (Tremblay, Barnes, & Cowie Bonne, 2014).

Furthermore, the success of the report cards and play-related physical activity interventions have also placed more attention on how children live and play in urban environments (e.g., increasingly driven to and from activities, fewer spaces to play freely outdoors), on the dominance of risk-aversion in western societies in which safety is placed above experience, on the growth and popularity of electronic devices for children, and, finally, on the academic pressures placed on children (Tremblay et al., 2014). In our book, we express caution and some concern with regard to such discourses and will address many of these in our upcoming chapters. In the outline of our theoretical perspectives in the next section, readers will be made aware of our critical approach in this book, and it will be more apparent as to why we are concerned with public health's incursions into play.

Theoretical perspectives

A Foucauldian approach to our research places emphasis on the critical examination of taken-for-granted assumptions and values underlying the expertise and health prescriptions targeting children, all of which are closely tied to the advancement of certain kinds of health behaviours and certain forms of play. Here we outline the main theoretical threads that have framed our research.

In his essay entitled "The politics of health in the eighteenth century" (Foucault, 1980), Michel Foucault describes how over the course of the 18th century the health of the population became a political objective, and that a medical authority developed which began to place rules and regulations on health and social life. This development was the result of the organisation of a politics of health (noso-politics), in which disease was seen as a political and economic problem. Through the exercise of power over economic regulations, public order and hygiene, health became an imperative for the population (Foucault, 1980). The economic rationalisation of health was a particularly important development of the 18th century and it continues to be manifest in contemporary health governance, for instance, in the way an "imperative of health" is placed on the population, and in this case children, with regard to their everyday lives and leisure practices.

Essential to the development of this form of governance was the reliance on expert knowledge. Turner (1997) writes that institutions with expertise such as the law, medicine or public health wielded increasing authority over the population, although the coercive nature of such institutions was disguised by their involvement in the problems of the population (i.e., birth and death rate, body weight, illness and so forth) for which they provided expert solutions. A set of "technologies of power", including the development of medicine, health surveillance, the production of norms for everything from intelligence to weight, to child development, and the self-regulatory practices to align one's behaviours with these norms, have become established components for governing life in modern industrialised societies (Petersen & Lupton, 1996). The authority held by health expertise is pertinent as it shapes the population's behaviour not by enforcing it, but by an overwhelming claim to truth and rationality (Lupton, 1995; Miller & Rose, 1990). As such, one might suggest that it is by relying on "truths" and "rational arguments" about childhood health, constructed through expert medical and public health advice, that issues such as childhood obesity and concerns about declining play have become central to public health action, and have facilitated justifications to intervene on children's leisure behaviours (Fullagar, 2009; McDermott, 2007). Drawing on Foucauldian theoretical concepts allows us to examine contemporary public health prescriptions, specifically around children's play, and to analyse how these rely on normative conceptions of childhood, health and leisure which have been constructed as "truths" through expert medical knowledge.

Biopower was a significant component of this new form of governmentality (Foucault, 1978, 1980, 2003, 2008) and included the efforts on the part of a state to solidify itself through the discipline of individual bodies and the regulation of the population in the name of productivity and health. While historically addressing adult health and productivity, children's health and leisure activities have also come to be subsumed in these efforts. For instance, children in contemporary industrialised societies are often conceived of as a population at risk of various ailments, most notably of obesity, and are thus viewed as requiring society-wide surveillance, measurement and regulation for establishing appropriate norms around their health and social activities (WHO, 2000, 2004, 2012a, 2012b). Children's bodies and their health-related activities are thus specific sites for public health action, and children are urged to self-regulate their behaviours to align with prescriptive norms. The concept of biopower is analytically useful for understanding how an "imperative of health" around children's leisure and play activities may be gaining authority precisely due to the medical knowledges surrounding childhood obesity and the urgency of its prevention.

Bringing together Foucault's concept of biopower and the idea of pedagogy as a "pedagogy of *bios*", Harwood (2009) has coined the concept of "biopedagogy". This biopedagogy aims to teach people about how to live, eat and generally how to behave in healthy ways (p. 15). Harwood (2009) argues that the growing concerns with children's obesity should be understood as linked to biopower and that the various practices promoting health within obesity discourses can be understood as biopedagogies of this biopower (p. 17). As an orienting theoretical concept, biopedagogies draws attention to both the disciplinary pedagogies directed at an individualised body (e.g., the child's body and his/her specific activities) as well as to regulatory strategies aimed at the population (e.g., children at risk of obesity) (Harwood, 2009). Burrows (2009) describes government programmes and health practices as biopedagogies aimed at families. She writes that state power is represented by government programmes and documents and operates through "a diffuse set of technologies to govern the actions of families, but also constitute families' understanding of themselves as viable, good and healthful" (p. 127). Biopedagogical analyses encourage the questioning of practices involved in obesity prevention, including the interrogation of the ways in which individuals are being informed through various programmes about how to be healthy citizens, as well as the examination of new norms that are being constructed around childhood obesity (Harwood, 2009). Furthermore, an examination of the practices and technologies used to govern behaviour is also central to an analysis of biopedagogies, as these work not only at the level of the material body (i.e., to shape bodies), but also work to produce subjects (i.e., the kinds of parents and children desired), their practices and beliefs (Burrows, 2009). Biopedagogies is therefore a valuable critical lens through which to concretely examine current interventions in Canadian public health (and other public health agencies across the globe) that address children's play as part of obesity discourses and to problematise the normalising and regulating practices that inform children and families about "how to play" properly.

As biopedagogies encourage individuals to change their lifestyles through various disciplinary techniques, they are also conceived as operating within the neo-liberal understanding of individuals as prudent and rational (Rail & Lafrance, 2009). Indeed, since the mid-20th century, there has been a sharp turn towards neo-liberal political economic practices, evidenced in the transformation of welfare states during the 1980s in countries such as the United States and the United Kingdom (Harvey, 2005), and premised on the belief that human well-being is best advanced by freeing up constraints on individual entrepreneurism and ensuring free markets through deregulation and privatisation (Harvey, 2005). This neo-liberal economic configuration has also come to shape modern public health approaches. Individuals are increasingly required to "assume responsibility for ensuring, monitoring, and acting upon their own health statuses" (Nadesan, 2008, p. 108) and are expected to live their lives in prudent and calculating ways, themselves monitoring and managing ever-present (and ever-increasing) health risks (Petersen & Lupton, 1996). Petersen (1997) has argued that the preventive techniques of health promotion reflect neo-liberal rationalities that target the "individual-as-enterprise" (p. 197); the individual who is expected to manage his/her own health in order to be productive, and to adhere to health norms through self-regulatory practices (Rose, 1999). An important element of a neo-liberal rationality is that individuals who become increasingly responsible for their own health and exposure to risk are also more willing to do so, as these self-governing actions come to be equated with personal fulfilment (Lupton, 1995; Miller & Rose, 1990). Under neo-liberalism, self-improvement becomes internalised "as a moral duty for one and all" (Rail, 2012, p. 24).

Much research, including the work in sociologies of childhood (Castañeda, 2002; James & James, 2004; Mayall, 1996; Mitchell & Reid-Walsh, 2002), youth surveillance studies (Dillabough & Kennelly, 2010; Gallagher & Fusco, 2006; Kirk, 1998; Giroux, 2004; Philo & Smith, 2003) and children's and youth's geographies (Aitken, 2001; Fusco,

2007, 2012; Holloway & Valentine, 2000; Katz, 1998; McKendrick, 1999; Valentine, 1996), all point towards the influence of economic neo-liberalization in the increased management, structuring and supervision of children's lives. According to Roberts (2016) and Zuzanek (2016), this includes the global restructuring of children's lives through an increased appetite for educational qualifications and the availability of new information and communication technologies as key moments in the refocusing on children's bodies and activities, with most countries resembling the west in articulations of youth and childhood. Indeed, in middle-class sectors, and now increasingly in working-class populations in western societies, forms of individualisation have taken hold (Roberts, 2016). This focus on the individual combined with the responsibility discourse of neo-liberalism has meant that every parent and child is deemed responsible for their own biographies, for planning their own futures (James & James, 2004; Roberts, 2016, p. 15) and for making sure they contribute effectively to economic competitiveness and efficiency (Furlong, 2012).

The way neo-liberal rationalities shape public health specifically is relevant as it underscores the ways in which families and children are currently being addressed with regard to the monitoring and managing of their health and social activities, and it highlights the economic rationale underlying many public health interventions geared at children. For instance, the authors in Dagkas and Burrows' (2016) book on families, youth and physical activity examine the diverse ways in which families relate to and take up imperatives around "education, health, sport and physical education" (p. 1). The book shows the range of "positionalities and experiences" (p. 2) that exist around notions of family, health pedagogy, physical education, sport and physical activity, and through such diverse accounts, they disrupt some of the dominant assumptions about these topics. In our case, the discourse on play is situated within the larger obesity discourse in which individuals (children, parents, families) are encouraged (prescribed) to monitor their behaviours in relation to dominant ideas about healthy exercise and diet (Rail, 2009).

This prompts us to question how public health practices are encouraging children and families to manage their risk of obesity (i.e., self-govern their lives) by adopting appropriately healthy ways of living, eating and even playing. Understanding the public health discourse around children's health and play as existing within neo-liberal forms of governing provides a frame for examining who is made responsible for children's appropriate, healthy or normal (dominant) forms of play, and for how children and their play activities may be considered economically important in the context of children's obesity prevention.

It is important to note of course that, historically, children's bodies, pleasures and recreational activities have also been subject to other kinds of regulations and scrutiny, particularly regarding sports and physical education (Baker, 2001; Green & Smith, 2016; Kirk, 1998), and this was relevant especially for middle-class children. However, once the arena of organised sport became increasingly available and popular for middle-class children, social attention turned towards managing play, recreation and sport opportunities for racially minoritised and economically disadvantaged communities (Frost, 2010). This was not always benevolent in nature. Rather, it was based on social control and aimed at reducing crime in urban areas through playgrounds/courts/recreation parks for young racialised boys and counter-culture ("at-risk") youth. For example, while the proliferation of midnight basketball leagues (Hartmann, 2016) and skateparks (Borden, 2001) have given young people the opportunity to play, these activities have also been critiqued because of their links to the surveillance and containment of so-called dangerous youth (Cole, 1996; Cole & Andrews, 2011). The containment of racialised and economically disadvantaged youth through sport and recreation has not changed much (Fleming, 2016), however contemporary neo-liberal discourses around children's play appear to be squarely directed at middle-class youth and their families (Wright & Macdonald, 2010).

Neo-liberalist discourses operate, paradoxically, alongside the *UN Convention on the Rights of the Child* (UNCRC) (1989), which aims to refocus attention on the rights of children to rest and leisure. The *UNCRC* highlights that it is important "to create time and space for children to engage in spontaneous recreation and creativity, and to promote societal attitudes that support and encourage such activity" (International Play Association, 2016, p. 1). The *International Play Association* writes, however, that:

> children's use of public space for play, recreation and their own cultural activities is impeded by the increasing commercialization and privatization of public areas, from which children are excluded or unwelcome.
>
> (2016, p. 3)

It is within these contexts that we weigh in with our theorisations of public health and play to examine how the increasing techno-rationalism of play in a neo-liberalist society is juxtaposed with the everyday narratives and experiences of children playing. Our discussion is also situated within ongoing debates around children's play: that children do not play enough, are not taking enough risks in play, are spending too much time on screens and are finding less and less pleasure in play activities. While there is a great deal more to be written about children, play, physical activity, sport and leisure, we hope that this book on public health and play contributes in some measure to the growing critical literature on childhood, play and socio-cultural life.

Methods and data collection[1]

The objectives and methods described in the following sections were those used to collect and analyse data for the PhD thesis research. The current book draws on the data collected for the PhD dissertation, but, as mentioned earlier, it also includes and integrates new academic and popular literature as well as media discussions and debates around childhood and play since 2014. This new literature updates the material around children's play in public health examined in the PhD dissertation, and it expands on the arguments made therein to include new and emerging topics on children's play as well as discussions of play from the perspectives of connected fields of research and practice, such as sports and physical education.

Objectives and approach

The PhD dissertation had three specific objectives regarding children's play and its entrance into public health discourse. The first objective was to identify the dominant positions, values, assumptions and practices underlying the public health discourse on children's play and to examine the ways in which this discourse privileges particular forms of play, while possibly obscuring others. As a second objective, the study explored children's own constructions of playing. As the final objective, it juxtaposed these two discourses on play to examine how the public health discourse shaped the meanings and affective experiences of playing for children. In order to address these inquiries, the dissertation placed particular emphasis on how the concept of "play" was constructed in two specific realms: first, within public health discourses and second, in children's photographs and narratives about their play. An emphasis was thus placed on *discourse*: on how it is constructed, and on how it shapes knowledge and understandings of children's play.

The analyses of dominant narratives, knowledges and practices underlying the public health discourse on children's play, as well as the examination of children's own discursive constructions of play, were positioned within social constructionist and post-structuralist perspectives. That is, the ideas that were generally understood to be "true" within public health literature regarding the constitution of a healthy child, a healthy weight or healthy forms of leisure were viewed as contingent concepts; they were viewed as providing only one possible conceptualisation of these notions informed by a particular socio-political, cultural and historical context. Critically examining these taken-for-granted understandings was important as they also informed the subject positions and identities available for children and shaped children's own constructions of play. The PhD research questions and approaches thus guided the methodological decisions taken to bring two qualitative components together: first a discourse analysis of public health texts that addressed children's play and second an examination of children's visual and narrative constructions of play. These two components were first examined individually and then juxtaposed and placed in dialogue with one another.

Discourse analysis

Taking a Foucauldian discourse analytical approach meant adopting a critical stance towards the relationship between the public health discourse on children's play, the practices that were emerging as part of this discourse, and the various effects this was having on children's play. This allowed us to highlight how public health identifies, constructs and gives shape to discussions addressing children's play, and to show how the public health discourse on play is embedded in political, social and historical processes, and is shaped by scientific knowledge and health messages. Importantly, it also helped underscore the way discourses and practices create particular subjects desired by public health institutions (i.e., active children, experts on play etc.).

We conducted a discourse analysis of public health documents and websites drawing on Foucauldian political scientist and post-structural theorist Carol Bacchi's (2009) approach to analysing discourse. Bacchi's (2009) approach suggests that while particular problem representations are elaborated in institutional discourses (e.g., the problem of inactive play), the presumption that those governing are simply reacting to problems that already exist "out there" in the world must be challenged. She argues that dominant problem representations address only one of many possible competing constructions of a particular problem. Furthermore, she writes that governmental institutions have a privileged position, and their ways of constructing and understanding problems often dominate and become constituted in legislation, reports and technologies used to govern (Bacchi, 2009). As such, she suggests that these problem constructions are especially in need of critical examination.

Following this approach, we broadly searched the websites of six prominent health-related Canadian organisations for documents and information relating to children's health, physical activity, obesity, leisure activities and play. We collected varied documents including informative webpages, downloadable reports, summary reports, workbooks for families and children as well as media releases and web campaigns. Materials made available or published between 2000 and 2012 were included as they reflected the recently developing discourse on play at the time.

Photography

To integrate children within the research project we drew on the sociology of childhood approach which implies the adoption of specific epistemological and methodological positions (Balen, Blyth, Calabretto, Horrocks, & Manby, 2006; Christensen, 2004; Darbyshire, MacDougall, & Schiller, 2005; Matthews, 2007; McNamee & Seymour, 2013): that children are competent social actors, that they are heterogeneous, and that childhood is characterised by plurality. This approach takes the view that research concerning children should be conducted with, as opposed to simply on, children, and that it should not "ignor(e) the views of children as active agents and 'key informants' in matters pertaining to their health and well-being" (Darbyshire et al., 2005, p. 419). This approach reinforces the necessity of giving voice to children's concerns and experiences (Corsaro, 2011; Darbyshire et al., 2005; Matthews, 2007; McNamee & Seymour, 2013) and views children as creative and social agents that "produce their own unique children's cultures while simultaneously contributing to the production of adult societies" (Corsaro, 2011, p. 4). For our research, this meant placing emphasis on a child's definition of an activity or situation (such as play) and acknowledging that children are active in constructing their own meanings of the world (Burr, 2003), in this case, their meanings of play.

Photographs were thus taken during child-led walks, which allowed children to choose the context and places of play that were relevant to them. We recruited 25 English- and French-speaking boys ($n = 10$) and girls ($n = 15$) aged 7 to 11 years from diverse neighbourhoods on the island of Montreal, Canada. At the time of the study, four children were 7 years old, nine children were 8 years old, seven children were 9 years old, two children were 10 years old, and three children were 11 years old.

We collected the photographic, interview and observational data over two meetings with each of the children in their family home. The first meeting included the child taking photographs of anything inside and outside the home that represented play. The six favourite photographs chosen by the child were printed for the second meeting, which took place approximately 2 weeks after the first and included an open-ended interview with the child about play, using the six printed photographs as the basis for conversation.[2]

Additional material for the book

In addition to the material collected and analysed for the Montreal-based study, for this book we collected material that included current debates in the media (i.e., TV, internet, newspapers, blogs and discussion groups), more recent public health literature (i.e., recently published report cards and scientific literature) and research conducted from within related health disciplines, such as sport and physical education. All of this material related specifically to children's changing freedoms, new perspectives on risk in play and debates around the permissions for children to play freely.

Outline of the chapters

Play theorist Brian Sutton-Smith has labelled the dominant trend in which play is instrumentalised for various productive ends a rhetoric of "play as progress" (1997). According to Sutton-Smith, within this modern rhetoric, the primary benefit of play is that children develop and learn productively through it. It is within this rhetoric of "play as progress" that we situate much of the recent public health discussions of children's play found in Chapter 2. One expression of this rhetoric of play as progress can be seen in the overall emphasis placed on play as productive for children's health and development, and specifically in the way it is becoming embedded in the emerging public health discourse around children's physical health. This has begun to reorient the discussions about children's play and leisure to focus on health promotion and obesity prevention. While the idea that play can be productive in general is not new (see the discussion in Chapter 2), the reorientation towards a productive health-focused form of play, we argue, *is* new and may change the way play is experienced for children. This transformation of play into a productive form of physical activity for children is elaborated in Chapter 3. The transformation of play for children towards an activity that is primarily valued for its health benefits implies that the pleasure inherent in children's play and leisure activities is also undergoing transformation. Play that is required to be physically active, healthy and safe becomes highly governed, including the forms of pleasure promoted as part of this play. Within this discourse, children and their play can thus be seen as navigating a fine line between pleasure and obligation.

Beginning with a historical account of the societal and then public health–enforced control of pleasure, in Chapter 4 we discuss this tenuous relationship between pleasure and obligation in play. By the second half of the 20th century, we see that new ways of playing emerged for children involving new technologies, all of which quickly gained in popularity. These changes were compounded by the increasing amount of time that children were spending playing indoors due to the assumption that keeping children indoors also kept them safe from outdoor risks as a "culture of fear" around childhood was perpetuated. However, the inundation of risk narratives around children's outdoor play was met with a countercurrent of criticism from within public health which argued that these forms of play – sedentary and predominantly screen-based – engendered *new* forms of physical health risks. While the earlier concerns about risk in play involved fears about children playing unsupervised in the streets, or not "playing the right way" when unsupervised, the new technological and mass-marketed play landscape began to generate new ways for children to play, and this was laden with new forms of risks. These ideas around risk in play are further developed in Chapter 5.

We conclude the book with Chapter 6, which includes a discussion of the most recent and emerging trends and debates around children's play, their health and their social lives more broadly. Trends we cover include the following: the growing attempts to quantify and measure free and active play, the continuing commodification of play and leisure activities, the tendency to harken back to a tradition or to past notions of play and to analyse contemporary children's play with a nostalgic lens and, finally, the globalisation of discourses and practices around play that originated and are predominant in the global north. We end the book optimistically, outlining a few current directions and initiatives taking into account some of the critiques presented in this book: attempts to create spaces that forefront children's and youth's play activities, making children visible and their diverse activities possible, without prescriptive intent.

Notes

1 For more details regarding the methods relating to the two components of the original PhD study, please refer to the following articles: Alexander, S. A., Frohlich, K. L., & Fusco, C. (2014). 'Active play may be lots of fun . . . but it's certainly not

frivolous': The emergence of active play as a health practice in Canadian public health. *Sociology of Health & Illness*, 36(8), 1188–1204 *and* Alexander, S. A., Frohlich, K. L., & Fusco, C. (2014). Problematizing 'Play for Health' discourses through children's photo-elicited narratives. *Qualitative Health Research*, 24(10), 1329–1341.

2 As part of the ethical approval the study received from the Université de Montréal (Canada), all of the children and their parents signed consent or assent forms before participating, which gave us the permission to use their interviews and photographs in any subsequent research publications, such as this book.

References

Active Healthy Kids Global Alliance. (2017). Retrieved August 2017 from www.activehealthykids.org

Aitken, S. (2001). *Geographies of young people: The morally contested spaces of identity*. London: Routledge.

Alexander, S. A., Frohlich, K. L., & Fusco, C. (2014). 'Active play may be lots of fun . . . but it's certainly not frivolous': The emergence of active play as a health practice in Canadian public health. *Sociology of Health & Illness*, 36(8), 1188–1204.

Alexander, S. A., Frohlich, K. L., & Fusco, C. (2014). Problematizing 'play for health' discourses through children's photo-elicited narratives. *Qualitative Health Research*, 24(10), 1329–1341.

Anchor, R. (1978). History and play: Johan Huizinga and his critics. *History and Theory*, 17(1), 63–93.

Atkinson, M. (2009). *Battleground sports* (Vol. 1 and 2). Westport, CT: Greenwood Press.

Azzarito, L., & Macdonald, D. (2016). Unpacking gender/sexuality/race/disability/social class to understand the embodied experiences of young people in physical culture. In K. Green & A. Smith (Eds.), *Routledge handbook of youth sport* (pp. 321–331). Oxon, UK: Routledge.

Bacchi, C. (2009). *Analysing policy: What's the problem represented to be?* Melbourne: Pearson Education.

Baker, B. M. (2001). *In perpetual motion: Theories of power, educational history and the child*. New York, NY: Peter Lang Publishing.

Balen, R., Blyth, E., Calabretto, H., Horrocks, C., & Manby, M. (2006). Involving children in health and social research: 'Human becomings' or 'active beings'? *Childhood*, 13, 29–48.

Borden, I. (2001). *Skateboarding, space and the city: Architecture and the body*. Oxford: BERG.

Brackenridge, C., Pitchford, A., Russell, K., & Nutt, G. (2007). *Child welfare in football: An exploration of children's welfare in the modern game*. London: Routledge.

Brown, S. (2009). *Play: How it shapes the brain, opens the imagination, and invigorates the soul*. Toronto: Penguin Group.

Burr, V. (2003). *Social constructionism* (2nd ed.). London: Routledge.

Burrows, L. (2009). Pedagogizing families through obesity discourse. In J. Wright & V. Harwood (Eds.), *Biopolitics and the 'Obesity Epidemic': Governing bodies*. New York, NY: Routledge.

Caillois, R. (1961). *Man, play, games* (M. Barash, Trans.). Urbana, IL: University of Illinois Press.

Castañeda, C. (2002). *Figurations: Child, bodies, worlds.* Durham, NC: Duke University Press.

Chouinard, M. A. (2006, November 9). Laissez jouer les enfants!: Sports et loisirs organisés prennent trop de place. *Le Devoir.* Retrieved February 2010 from www.ledevoir.com/

Christensen, P. H. (2004). Children's participation in ethnographic research: Issues of power and representation. *Children and Society, 18,* 165–176.

Chudacoff, H. P. (2007). *Children at play: An American history.* New York, NY: New York University Press.

Cole, C. L. (1996). American Jordan: P.L.A.Y., consensus & punishment. *Sociology of Sport Journal, 13,* 336–397.

Cole, C. L., & Andrews, D. L. (2011). America's new son: Tiger Woods and America' multiculturalism. In D. Leonard & C. R. King (Eds.), *Commodified and criminalized: New racism and African Americans in contemporary sports* (pp. 23–40). Lanham, MD: Rowman & Littlefield.

Cordes, K. (2013). *Applications for recreation and leisure: For today and the future* (4th ed.). Urbana, IL: Sagamore Publishing.

Corsaro, W. A. (2011). *The sociology of childhood* (3rd ed.). London: Sage Publications.

Crawford, R. (1980). Healthism and the medicalization of everyday life. *International Journal of Health Services, 10*(3), 365–388.

Crawford, R. (2006). Health as a meaningful social practice. *Health: An Interdisciplinary Journal for the Social Study of Health, Illness and Medicine, 10*(4), 401–420.

Dagkas, S., & Armour, K. (2012). *Inclusion and exclusion through youth sport.* London: Routledge.

Dagkas, S., & Burrows, L. (Eds.). (2016). *Families, young people, physical activity and health: Critical perspectives.* London: Routledge.

Darbyshire, P., MacDougall, C., & Schiller, W. (2005). Multiple methods in qualitative research with children: More insight or just more? *Qualitative Research, 5*(4), 417–436.

Dillabough, J.-A., & Kennelly, J. (2010). *Lost youth in the global city: Class, culture and the Urban imaginary.* New York, NY: Routledge.

Dowling, F., Fitzgerald, H., & Flintoff, A. (2012). *Equity and difference in physical education, youth sport and health: A narrative approach.* London: Routledge.

Eichberg, H. (2017). *Questioning play: What play can tell us about social life.* London: Routledge.

Elkind, D. (2007). *The power of play: How spontaneous, imaginative activities lead to happier, healthier children.* Berkeley, CA: Da Capo Press.

Evans, J., Davis, B., & Wright, J. (2004). *Body knowledge and control: Studies in the sociology of physical education and health.* New York, NY: Routledge.

Evans, J., Rich, E., Davis, B., & Allwood, R. (2008). *Education, disordered eating and obesity discourse: Fat fabrications.* Oxon, UK: Routledge.

Fleming, S. (2016). Youth sport, race and ethnicity. In K. Green & A. Smith (Eds.), *Routledge handbook of youth sport* (pp. 287–296). Oxon, UK: Routledge.

Foucault, M. (1978). *History of sexuality: An introduction* (Vol. I). Toronto: Random House of Canada.
Foucault, M. (1980). The politics of health in the eighteenth century. In C. Gordon (Ed.), *Power/knowledge: Selected interviews and other writings 1972–1977*. New York, NY: Pantheon Books.
Foucault, M. (2003). *'Society must be defended': Lectures at the Collège de France, 1975–1976* (D. Macey, Trans.). New York, NY: Picador.
Foucault, M. (2008). *The birth of biopolitics: Lectures at the Collège de France 1978–1979* (G. Burchell, Trans.). New York, NY: Palgrave Macmillan.
Frost, J. L. (2010). *A history of children's play and play environments: Toward a contemporary child-saving movement*. New York, NY: Routledge.
Fullagar, S. (2009). Governing healthy family lifestyles through discourses of risk and responsibility. In J. Wright & V. Harwood (Eds.), *Biopolitics and the 'Obesity Epidemic': Governing bodies*. New York, NY: Routledge.
Furlong, A. (2012). *Youth studies: An introduction*. London: Routledge.
Fusco, C. (2007). Healthification and the promises of urban space: A textual analysis of representations of place, activity, youth (PLAY-ing) in the city. *International Review for the Sociology of Sport, 423*, 43–63.
Fusco, C. (2012). Moral geographies, healthification and neo-liberal urban imaginaries. In D. Andrews & M. Silk (Eds.), *Sport and neoliberalism: Politics, consumption, and culture* (pp. 143–159). Philadelphia, PA: Temple University Press.
Fusco, C., Moola, F., Faulkner, G., Buliung, R., & Richichi, V. (2012). Toward an understanding of children's perceptions of their transport geographies: (Non)active school travel and visual representations of the built environment. *Journal of Transport Geography, 20*(1), 62–70.
Gagen, E. (2000). Playing the part: Performing gender in America's playgrounds. In S. Holloway & G. Valentine (Eds.), *Children's geographies: Playing, living, learning* (pp. 213–229). London: Routledge.
Gallagher, K., & Fusco, C. (2006). I.D.ology and the technologies of public (school) space: An ethnographic inquiry into the neo-liberal tactics of social (re)production. *Journal of Ethnography and Education, 1*(3), 301–318.
Gard, M., & Wright, J. (2005). *The obesity epidemic: Science, morality and ideology*. New York, NY: Routledge.
Gatz, M., Messner, M. A., & Ball-Rokeach, S. J. (Eds.). (2002). *Paradoxes of youth and sport*. Albany, NY: State University of New York Press.
Giroux, H. (2004). *The terror of neoliberalism: Authoritarianism and the eclipse of democracy*. Boulder, CO: Paradigm.
Green, K., & Smith, A. (Eds.). (2016). *Routledge handbook of youth sport*. Oxon, UK: Routledge.
Gruneau, R. (2010). Trends in community sport participation and community sport organizations since the 1990s: Implications for West Vancouver. *Centre for sport policy studies working paper series, no. 3*. Toronto, OH: Centre for Sport Policy Studies, Faculty of Physical Education and Health, University of Toronto.
Gutman, M., & de Coninck-Smith, N. (2008). *Designing modern childhoods: History, space, and the material culture of children*. New Brunswick: Rutgers University Press.
Harper, S. (2009). *Lost adventures of childhood*. Original Documentary. Toronto, Canada: CTV.

Hartmann, D. (2016). *Midnight basketball: Race, sports and neoliberal social policy*. Chicago, IL: Chicago University Press.

Harvey, D. (2005). *A brief history of neoliberalism*. Oxford: Oxford University Press.

Harvey, S., & Light, S. (2013). *Ethics in youth sport: Policy and pedagogical applications*. London: Routledge.

Harwood, V. (2009). Theorizing biopedagogies. In J. Wright & V. Harwood (Eds.), *Biopolitics and the 'Obesity Epidemic': Governing bodies* (pp. 15–30). New York, NY: Routledge.

Holloway, S., & Valentine, G. (2000). *Children's geographies: Playing, living, learning*. London: Routledge.

Holt, N. (Ed.). (2008). *Positive youth development through sport*. Oxon, UK: Routledge.

Honoré, C. (2009). *Under pressure: Putting the child back in childhood*. Toronto: Random House.

Huizinga, J. (1949). *Homo Ludens: A study of the play-element in culture*. London: Routledge & Kegan.

Human Kinetics. (2013). *Introduction to recreation and leisure* (2nd ed.). Urbana Champaign, IL: Human Kinetics.

International Play Association (IPA). (2016). *Children's right to play and the environment – IPA discussion paper for UNCRC day of discussion 2016*. Retrieved July 2017 from http://ipaworld.org/childrens-right-to-play-and-the-environment/

James, A., & James, A. (2004). *Constructing childhood: Theory, policy, practice*. London: Palgrave MacMillian.

Jeske Crane, C. (2014, November 3). *Why kids are dropping out of organized sports*. Retrieved January 2018 from www.parentscanada.com/school/why-kids-are-dropping-out-of-organized-sports

Kamphorst, T., & Roberts, K. (1989). *Trends in sports: A multinational perspective*. Voorthuizen, The Netherlands: Giordano Bruno Culemborg.

Katz, C. (1998). Disintegrating developments: Global economic structuring and the eroding ecologies of youth. In T. Skelton & G. Valentine (Eds.), *Cool places: Geographies of youth cultures* (pp. 130–144). London: Routledge.

Kehler, M., & Atkinson, M. (2010). *Boys bodies: Speaking the unspoken*. New York, NY: Peter Lang.

Kennedy, P. (Writer). (2009). *The hurried infant: CBC ideas*. Toronto, Canada: Canadian Broadcasting Corporation (CBC).

Kirk, D. (1998). *Schooling bodies: School practice and public discourse, 1880–1950*. London: Leicester University Press.

Kremer, J., Trew, K., & Ogle, S. (Eds.). (1997). *Young people's involvement in sport*. London: Routledge.

Lang, M., & Harthill, M. (2015). *Safeguarding, child protection and abuse in sport: International perspectives in research, policy and practice*. Oxon, UK: Routledge.

Lester, S., & Russell, W. (2014). Turning the world upside down: Playing as the deliberate creation of uncertainty. *Children, 1*, 241–260. doi:10.3390/children1020241

Lupton, D. (1995). *The imperative of health: Public health and the regulated body*. London: Sage Publications.

Matthews, S. H. (2007). A window on the 'new' sociology of childhood. *Sociology Compass, 1*(1), 322–334.

Mayall, B. (1996). *Children, Health and the Social Order*. Buckingham: Open University Press.

McDermott, L. (2007). A governmental analysis of children 'at risk' in a world of physical inactivity and obesity epidemics. *Sociology of Sport Journal, 24*, 302–324.

McDonald, B. (Writer). (2009). *Getting serious about play*. Quirks and Quarks. Toronto, Canada: Canadian Broadcasting Corporation (CBC).

McKendrick, J. (1999). Playgrounds in the built environment. *Built Environment, 24*, 1–6.

McNamee, S., & Seymour, J. (2013). Towards a sociology of 10–12 year olds? Emerging methodological issues in the 'new' social studies of childhood. *Childhood, 20*(2), 156–168.

Messner, M. (2011). Gender ideologies, youth sports, and the production of soft essentialism. *Sociology of Sport Journal, 28*, 151–170.

Meyer, I. H., & Schwartz, S. (2000). Social issues as public health: Promise and peril. *American Journal of Public Health, 90*(8), 1189–1191.

Miller, P., & Rose, N. (1990). Governing economic life. *Economy and Society, 19*(1), 1–31.

Mitchell, C., & Reid-Walsh, J. (2002). *Researching children's popular culture: The cultural spaces of childhood*. New York, NY: Routledge.

Moore, R. (1987). Streets as playgrounds. In Moudon, A. (ed.), *Public streets for public use* (pp. 45–62). New York: Van Nostrand Rhinehold.

Nadesan, M. (2008). *Governmentality, biopower, and everyday life*. New York, NY: Routledge.

Parker, A., & Vinson, D. (2013). *Youth sport, physical activity and play: Policy, intervention and participation*. London: Routledge.

Petersen, A. (1997). Risk, governance and the new public health. In A. Petersen & R. Bunton (Eds.), *Foucault, health and medicine* (pp. 189–206). New York, NY: Routledge.

Petersen, A., & Lupton, D. (1996). *The new public health: Health and self in the age of risk*. London: Sage Publications.

Philo, C., & Smith, F. (2003). Guest editorial: Political geographies of children and young people. *Space and Polity, 7*, 99–115.

Rail, G. (2009). Canadian youth's discursive constructions of health in the context of obesity discourse. In J. Wright & V. Harwood (Eds.), *Biopolitics and the obesity "Epidemic": Governing bodies* (pp. 141–156). New York, NY: Routledge.

Rail, G. (2012). The birth of the obesity clinic: Confessions of the flesh, biopedagogies and physical culture. *Sociology of Sport Journal, 29*(2), 227–253.

Rail, G., & Lafrance, M. (2009). Confessions of the flesh and biopedagogies: Discursive constructions of obesity on Nip/Tuck. *Medical Humanities, 35*, 76–79.

Read, J. (2011). Gutter to garden: Historical discourses of risk in interventions in working class children's street play. *Children & Society, 25*(6), 421–434. doi:10.1111/j.1099-0860.2010.00293.x

Reinhart, R. (2014). Anhedonia and alternative sports. *Staps, 2*(104), 9–21.

Roberts, K. (2016). Young people and social change. In K. Green & A. Smith (Eds.), *Routledge handbook of youth sport* (pp. 10–17). Oxon, UK: Routledge.

Rose, N. (1999). *Governing the soul: The shaping of the private self* (2nd ed.). London: Free Association Books.

Skrabanek, P. (1994). *The death of humane medicine and the rise of coercive healthism*. The Social Affairs Unit. Bury St Edmunds, Suffolk: St Edmundsbury Press.

Skrabanek, P. (1994). *The death of humane medicine and the rise of coercive medicine*. Bury St Edmunds, Suffolk: St Edmundsbury Press.

Stearns, P. N. (2005). *Growing up: The history of childhood in a global context*. Waco, TX: Baylor University Press.

Strashin, J. (2016, May 10). *No more joiners: Why kids are dropping out of sports: Focus on elite athletes may drive others away, say experts studying decline of sports participation*. Retrieved January 2018 from www.cbc.ca/sports/sports-participation-canada-kids-1.3573955

Sutton-Smith, B. (1981). *A history of children's play: New Zealand, 1840–1950*. Philadelphia, PA: University of Pennsylvania Press.

Sutton-Smith, B. (1997). *The ambiguity of play*. Boston, MA: Harvard University Press.

Sydnor, S., & Fagan, R. (2012). Plotlessness, ethnography, ethology: Play. *Cultural Studies ↔ Critical Methodologies*, 12(1), 72–81.

Thompson, S. (1999). *Mother's taxi: Sport and women's labour*. New York, NY: SUNY.

Thorpe, H. (2012). 'Sex, drugs, and snowboarding': (Il)legitimate definitions of taste and lifestyle in a physical youth culture. *Leisure Studies*, 3(1), 31–51.

Torkildsen, G. (2005). *Leisure and recreation management* (5th ed.). Oxon, UK: Routledge.

Tremblay, M., Barnes, J., & Cowie Bonne, J. (2014). Impact of the active healthy kids Canada report card: A 10-year analysis. *Journal Physical Act Health*, 1, S3–S20.

Turner, B. S. (1997). Foreword: From governmentality to risk, some reflections on Foucault's contribution to medical sociology. In A. Petersen & R. Bunton (Eds.), *Foucault, health and medicine* (pp. ix–xxi). New York, NY: Routledge.

United Nations. (1989). *Convention on the rights of the child*. Retrieved July 2017 from www.ohchr.org/en/professionalinterest/pages/crc.aspx

Valentine, G. (1996). Angels and devils: Moral landscapes of childhood. *Environment and Planning D: Society and Space*, 14, 581–599.

Wenner, M. (2009, January 28). The serious need for play: Free, imaginative play is crucial for normal social, emotional and cognitive development. It makes us better adjusted, smarter and less stressed. *Scientific American Mind*.

Whitehead, J., Telfer, H., & Lambert, J. (2014). *Values in youth sport and physical education*. London: Routledge.

WHO. (2000). *Obesity: Preventing and managing the global epidemic*. Geneva, Switzerland: World Health Organization.

WHO. (2004). *Obesity: Preventing and managing the global epidemic*. Geneva, Switzerland: World Health Organization.

WHO. (2012a). *Global strategy on diet, physical activity and health*. Geneva, Switzerland: World Health Organization.

WHO. (2012b). *Population-based approaches to childhood obesity prevention*. Geneva, Switzerland: World Health Organisation.

Wright, J., & Harwood, V. (2009). *Biopolitics and the 'Obesity Epidemic': Governing bodies*. New York, NY: Routledge.

Wright, J., & Macdonald, D. (2010). *Young people, physical activity and the everyday*. London: Routledge.

Zuzanek, J. (2016). Youth's use of time from comparative, historical and developmental perspectives. In K. Green & A. Smith (Eds.), *Routledge handbook of youth sport* (pp. 26–41). Oxon, UK: Routledge.

Chapter 2

Playing as progress

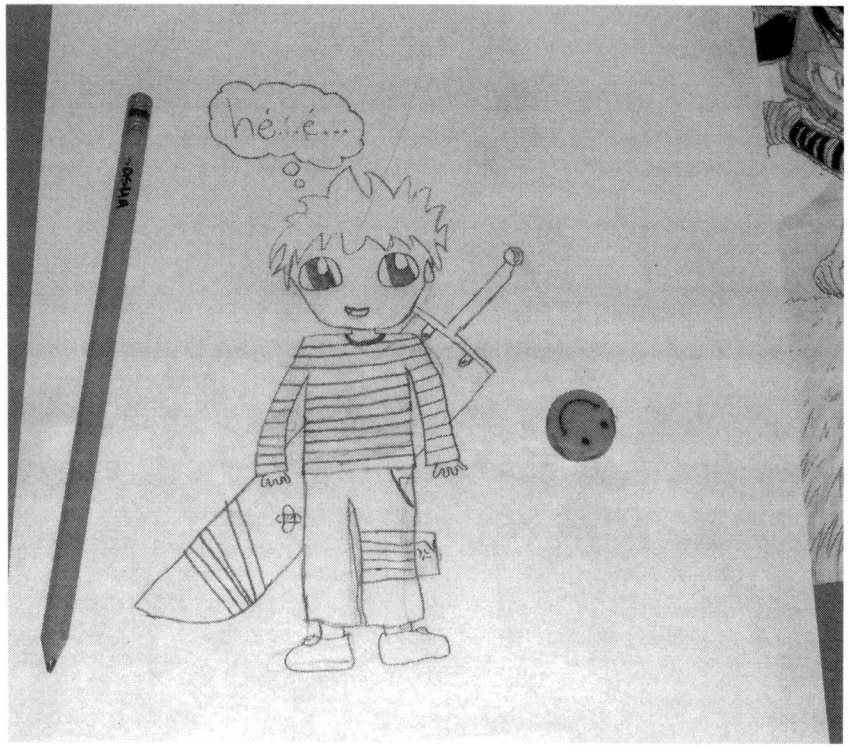

Figure 2.1 Sébastien (11 years old) took a photo of his drawing.

Introduction

> Work consists of whatever a body is obliged to do. Play consists of whatever a body is not obliged to do.
> (Mark Twain, *The Adventures of Tom Sawyer*)

Unlike the kind of play described in the Mark Twain quotation, in which playing is an activity one is "not obliged to do", playing today has increasingly been set to a schedule, is spatially and temporally circumscribed, and is frequently goal-directed (i.e., through play dates, "time to play", recess breaks and designated play spaces or playgrounds). Current trends in children's play indeed differ from historical accounts of play. As Frost (2010) suggests:

> play throughout history was relatively free, intertwined with work, spontaneous, and set in the playgrounds of the wilderness, fields, streams and barnyards. Children in cities enjoyed similar forms of play, but their playgrounds were the vacant lands, parks and surrounding countryside or seashore.
>
> (p. 1)

This chapter provides a historical lens on children's play to help understand how playing has come to be increasingly structured and productive. We provide an account of the way play has historically been discussed, how it has come to be instrumentalised over time, and how the idea of productive and efficient play emerged. In the first section of this chapter, we trace some of the literature that began to endorse children's play as a foundation for their emotional and social well-being, as well as research suggesting that playing is inextricably linked to the advancement of education and to children's optimal development. In parallel, we discuss the movement that advocated for play as a way to improve physical strength. Through this we show how discussions and early studies about play have historically shaped where, with whom, when and with what goals children were encouraged to play. An historical understanding of these areas of research is important as a way to identify the dominant discourses that frame contemporary discussions about children's play, and also to appreciate the social and cultural importance attributed to children's play today. Particularly relevant is that this work collectively forms the basis for growing concerns about what is called the disappearance of children's play, and the interventions to protect and promote children's play today. In the second section of this chapter we address the contemporary perspectives on play, specifically a rhetoric of "play as progress" that surrounds discussions about the importance of play, and the ways in which play is encouraged for the development of particular kinds of citizens, in this case, active and healthy child citizens.

Historical perspectives

Playing for psychological, educational and physical development

Psychologists generally, and developmental psychologists especially, have long been at the forefront of discussions about childhood and children's play, and in studying and advocating for the central importance of play for children's overall development (Chudacoff, 2007). Since at least the 16th century, as outlined by Boekhoven (2009) and Baker (2001), there have been changes in attitudes and discourses around the "child" in Europe and in North America as illustrated in the writings of philosophers, psychologists and historians (e.g., John Locke, Jean-Jacques Rousseau, G. Stanley Hall, Philippe Ariès) (Baker, 2001). As Baker (2001) suggests, each era viewed the child through a different lens with a "shifting conceptualization of the child, power, and strategies for education-rearing" (p. 3) and thus also shifting "truths" and assertions about the imaginary of "the child". For instance, in 16th-century North America, a strict approach was taken towards child-rearing, specifically with regard to children's "moral well-being" (Boekhoven, 2009, p. 3). Children were viewed as being sinful, and the Protestant work ethic of strict discipline was intended to protect children, promote wholesome and purposeful activities, while denying activities that were deemed frivolous (i.e., play) (Boekhoven, 2009). Boekhoven suggests that our contemporary focus on sports and organised leisure activities for children emerged from this thinking.

Later, during the Industrial Revolution of the 18th and 19th centuries, and due to the advent of universal schooling for children, there were changes in the amount of time, space and attention dedicated to children (Boekhoven, 2009). A new understanding of childhood emerged during this period, in which children were no longer viewed as being simply small adults but were seen as progressing through a specific developmental period: childhood (Boekhoven, 2009; Postman, 1994). Due in part to the growing interest in childhood as a developmental phase, the 19th to mid-20th centuries were characterised by increasing expert knowledge about childhood development and child-rearing in the fields of psychology and education (Lupton, 1995; Nadesan, 2010; Reiger, 1985; Turmel, 2008). Scientific developments and societal changes informed the psychological interest in children's development and contributed to a growing preoccupation with what Turmel (2008) has termed the "nascent science of childhood" (p. 3). A new attitude toward children developed along with a new importance placed on this distinct phase of childhood and the concern for providing children with appropriate direction (Chudacoff, 2007; Rose, 1999; Turmel, 2008). The late 19th and early 20th century interest in standardisation, classification, data collection and statistical thinking around childhood development in North America thus also led to the emergence of the notion of "normalcy" which strongly shaped the study of childhood and child psychology (Turmel, 2008). New psychological expertise played a significant role in helping to construct the idea of what we consider to be a normal child and of what normal childhood development constituted. For instance, Turmel (2008) writes:

> developmental standards, which are produced at the same time through technologies of regulation, bring about three different forms of normalcy: the normal child as average, as healthy and as acceptable.
> (Turmel, 2008, p. 13)

Late 19th- and early 20th-century research in the field of child development and psychology (i.e., Jean Piaget, 1896–1980, Switzerland; Lev Vygotsky, 1896–1934, Russia) led to a burgeoning interest in research on children's play, specifically as it became increasingly viewed as an integral part of childhood cognitive development (Boekhoven, 2009; Smith & Pellegrini, 2005). In many industrialising countries (e.g., USA, France, England, Australia), medical, psychological and education professionals were celebrating the new "age of childhood" (Nadesan, 2010; Reiger, 1985; Turmel, 2008); children were becoming "objects of serious study" and their learning and play activities were increasingly moved "under the magnifying glass" (Chudacoff, 2007, p. 72) in order to understand their role for childhood development.

This new importance attributed to childhood and its study also led to a new acceptability of, and a new value attributed to, children's play. Unlike the historically stricter views about childhood, in the late 19th century more permissive child-centred attitudes towards playing developed, and the research fields of child studies and psychology began to advocate for children to use their "play instinct" to develop their own "play culture" (Chudacoff, 2007, p. 92).

Children's play in western industrialised societies has, since then, not only been considered synonymous with childhood, but as it was increasingly the domain of psychologists and educational reformers, play came to be seen as a critical component of children's overall development (Chudacoff, 2007). American historian Howard Chudacoff (2007) writes that already in 1896 psychologist T. R. Croswell, who conducted a survey with 2,000 children about their play preferences, argued that "free, unstructured play – as distinct from work or school and taking place without strict adult interference – had beneficial effects" (Chudacoff, 2007, p. 92). In this sense, the developmental value that was being attributed to play meant it was already being instrumentalised: play was increasingly considered important and viewed as requiring protection and promotion because of its cognitive benefits for children.

Furthermore, the belief that children's play was critical for academic learning was also advanced by early pioneers of childhood education, such as Friedrich Froebel (1782–1852, Germany), Maria Montessori (1870–1952, Italy/Netherlands), and Rudolph Steiner (1861–1925, Croatia/Switzerland), the founders of the Montessori and Waldorf schools in the late 19th century (Pellegrini, 1995; Read, 2006; Roskos & Christie, 2001; Santer, Griffiths, & Goodall, 2007). The idea of play as an educational activity emerged together with the commitment to valuing play only if it was considered useful (Chudacoff, 2007). The new appreciation of children's play was thus also imbued with the desire to regulate play to promote academic learning. For instance, in the United States, growing numbers of child-rearing experts advocated for playing with blocks and games as educational, while advice manuals about child-rearing and appropriate forms of play were being published in numerous countries (Nadesan, 2010; Read, 2011; Reiger, 1985; Rose, 1999).

In the United States and England, new play materials were produced for developmental purposes; educational games, toys and healthy play guidelines were encouraged for the optimally developing "virtuous middle-class child" (Chudacoff, 2007, p. 44). Chudacoff (2007) writes that the educational function of toys emerged from a middle-class "aspiration for self-improvement" (p. 117) and as such, while toys were viewed as being fun, they were more importantly increasingly seen as instrumental for intellectual development (Chudacoff, 2007; Rose, 1999). Indeed, middle-class American parents of the late 19th century began to mistrust play or toys that were considered merely frivolous and which "stirred utter fantasy" (Chudacoff, 2007, p. 83), preferring toys that would "impart useful skills" (p. 83) and those that would contribute to "wholesome exercise" (p. 83). Toward the mid- to late 20th century, play was frequently explicitly promoted for productive purposes, for instance, to "combine supervised play with supervised education to make schools 'fun'" (Chudacoff, 2007, p. 165). The growth and popularity of organisations such as the YMCA and sports gymnasiums created a space for organised play where working-class children were recruited to learn middle-class values of "teamwork, fair play and accomplishment" (Chudacoff, 2007, p. 115).

Social and health regulation: confining and controlling play

According to Frost (2010), in the late 19th and early 20th centuries, two parallel play and playground movements emerged that shaped the trends for children's play today and that related to the confinement and control of children's play for social benefits and health promotion. These trends originated in two places and at two points in time; the latter half of the 19th century in Germany and the American play and playground movement beginning near the turn of the 20th century. The former, emerging in parallel in several countries, emphasised the health and fitness benefits of vigorous outdoor exercise. It was based initially on the German physical fitness tradition, emphasising physical development and recreation. It was documented and substantiated amongst others by the esteemed German doctor and micro-biologist Robert Koch (1843–1910, Germany). The main purpose of this movement was to counteract the harmful effects of city life and its growing demands by emphasising physical fitness, which expanded to include sports and recreation. Frost (2010) suggests that the heritage of the German physical fitness tradition lives on today in the United States through the National Recreation and Park Association (NRPA), which champions physical fitness with a stress on safety. Its main audience was urban recreation and park professionals, and its emphasis on physical development and safety has made its mark on playground design and standards.

The American play and playground movement, on the other hand, was influenced by the child study movement and was partially centred in child research stations at major American universities during the early 1900s. Indeed, it was during the early 1900s that the child-saving movement phased into a child study movement. Leading educators and psychologists ushered in a scientific era that led to the eventual establishment of research centres on childhood, on play, as well as the formation of nursery schools and kindergartens based on principles of child development and including new play environments designed to facilitate children's wide range of play forms.

The development of Kindergartens in Germany would also formalise the term "playground" and popularise ideas about, and links between, playing, psychological well-being and learning. Friedrich Froebel, the architect of the kindergarten, opened his first kindergarten in Bad Blankenburg, Germany in 1840. Of play he wrote:

> Play is the purest, most spiritual activity of man at this stage, and, at the same time, typical of human life as a whole – of the inner hidden

natural life in man and all things. It gives, therefore, joy, freedom, contentment, inner and outer rest, peace with the world. It holds the source of all that is good. . . . Play at this time is of deep significance . . . the germinal leaves of all later life.

(Fröbel, 1887, pp. 54–55, cited in Frost, 2010, p. 6)

Froebel's playgrounds were in nature and in gardens established on schoolyards and it was in these more confined spaces that children played. These playgrounds were in many ways different from the country surroundings and farms where most children lived, and they offered specific times for play during the day – recesses – and were considered rich places for learning.

At the same time as Froebel's playground initiatives, then, the conduct of play and the development of playgrounds were guided by the child study movement and new developments in childhood psychology. For instance, play advocates of the child study movement wanted to ensure that children's play was increasingly under parental control, either in the home or at an adult-supervised playground, and outdoor spaces for play in playgrounds were confined to precise areas for the easy supervision of safe play (Chudacoff, 2007). Members of the American child study movement were warning of the dangers of unsupervised street play, and mothers were being advised that it was their responsibility to ensure their child's safety when he/she was not in school by, for instance, "encouraging [them] to be involved in youth groups and supervised playground activities" (Chudacoff, 2007, p. 106).

Chudacoff (2007) suggests that what concerned child study experts in the early 20th century most was that city children were not "using their time out of school and away from parental supervision in approved ways – in a word, they were 'idling'" (p. 109). As such, as Frost (2010) writes, the institutionalisation of play began to harden during the early 1900s when community and government groups began to provide for all ages and to institute year-round play organisations (activities that parents will recognise today as the constant demands to keep children busy). Indeed, while in the early decades of the 20th century few American children were involved in after-school or summer programmes involving "lessons, leagues, clubs, and camps" (Chudacoff, 2007, p. 100), by the mid-twentieth century the growth of playgrounds, schoolyards, organised sports and educational games had the aims of regulating children's play and of specifically preparing children for later life (Chudacoff, 2007; Hart, 2002).

Similar to the child study movement, the playground movement was also influenced by modern trends toward standardisation and efforts to structure play, and in this case, structured play on supervised, well-equipped playgrounds owned by municipal governments. One purpose of the standardisation of playgrounds was to institutionalise provisions for play and to organise play experiences, and a second purpose was the application of modern psychological and biological theories for improving cognitive skills, moral tendencies and instilling social values through play experiences (Frost, 2010; Kozlovsky, 2008). The movement to institutionalise play grew gradually during the early 1900s when community and government groups began to provide for all ages and to institute year-round play organisation (Frost, 2010, p. 103). Frost (2010) writes that as play leaders were trained, they were sent into public playgrounds and into the streets to mark off play zones, supplement the limited number of public playgrounds and organise and supervise children's play (p. 103).

Some of the reforms of the early child-saving movement (later child study movement) were also intertwined with the growth of other organisations for the shaping of modern children's play and playgrounds. For instance, alongside the *Playground Association of America* and the *American Playground Movement*, there were numerous reforms and sub-movements to create children's museums, school gardens, nature study, botanical gardens and summer camps. The *Playground Association of America* was responsible for building thousands of city parks and playgrounds, primarily focused on the idea of the German physical fitness movement (Frost, 2010).

Linked to all of the efforts around play structuring and organisation was the perception emerging at the same time in North America, the UK, Australia and other European countries that there were fewer opportunities for children to play outdoors freely (Gutman & de Coninck-Smith, 2008). In the 19th century, public spaces in English and American cities, including streets and sidewalks, were a relatively common play space for working-class children (Chudacoff, 2007; Hart, 2002; Read, 2011). These children did not have access to private play areas and thus took over public spaces to create a play culture for themselves in the streets of the urban outdoors (Chudacoff, 2007; Read, 2011). However, in the late 19th and early 20th centuries, outdoor play changed through growing interventions on children's street play.

For instance, Read (2011) examined the developments and transformations around children's street play in 19th- and 20th-century England. She argues that the views towards street play were strongly shaped by the child-saving movement and the development of free kindergartens for poor children. "Gutter play", as "street play" was called, was considered risky for working-class children, and was seen as a "conduit for filth, both physical and moral, and thus embodied threat, both to children and society" (Read, 2011, p. 1). Aimed primarily at working-class children believed to be inappropriately socialised and thus unfamiliar with "appropriately moral" ways of playing (Hart, 2002, p. 138), expert reformers taught children about the proper ways to play (Read, 2011). The aim was to relocate "gutter children" "within the healthy, neo-rural and, crucially, morally improving play space provided by the free kindergarten" (Read, 2011, p. 4). Middle-class and upper-class children, for their part, were discouraged from playing with working-class children in order to prevent them from adopting their less savoury forms of play (Chudacoff, 2007; Hart, 2002; Read, 2011). Read (2011) cites the founder of the Michaelis Free Kindergarten: "[w]e must go into the streets and show the children how to play" (Read, 2011, p. 7).

Hart's (2002) research on the playground movement in early 20th-century New York similarly suggests that playgrounds developed in part out of a concern that playing in the streets, particularly for immigrant children, would be a risk for their health and safety, and that these street-playing children were becoming a threat to society (Hart, 2002). Hart (2002) writes that in large part, playgrounds were created as a way of getting children off the street; "away from bad influences and under the control of known socializing agents" (p. 138). Sutton-Smith (1997), who has also commented on the historical function of playgrounds and organised play, suggests that in the second half of the twentieth century there were growing attempts to:

> "domesticate" children through the introduction of playgrounds and playground equipment, organized sports, fenced-in school yards, organized clubs (Scouts), recreation (dancing, gymnastics), and supervision of play.
>
> (p. 121)

As such, a new form of adult-guided or prescribed play was developed to encourage appropriate child behaviours through interventions on play, the growth of kindergartens and the creation of confined play spaces such as playgrounds. Certainly, by the early to mid-twentieth century in many industrialised countries, playgrounds, and the development of sports clubs, as well as the general discouragement of street play had changed the atmosphere of outdoor play for children. The belief that children had to be protected from an increasingly complex society (i.e., growth in industrialisation, urbanisation, immigration), brought to the forefront concerns about outdoor play for children (Chudacoff, 2007; Gutman & de Coninck-Smith, 2008; Hart, 2002). The urban outdoors were increasingly considered too dangerous for children's play (Gutman & de Coninck-Smith, 2008; Nadesan, 2010). For instance, Rivkin (1997) writes about the development of large-scale urbanisation and industrialization that "deprived children of outdoor, in particular nature based, experiences" (p. 61) due to a growing reliance on cars in cities. This, together with children's increasing institutionalisation (i.e., in schools, childcare, organised sports, lessons etc.), was perceived as impacting children's outdoor exploration and the range of spaces in which children could play greatly diminished (Rivkin, 1997).

Given these changes to, and confinements of, children's play, it is not surprising that Karsten (2005) found that children in Amsterdam experienced what she has called a "shrinking territory" for play (p. 276) between 1950 and 2005, especially due to changes in their freedom of movement. She writes that public areas in the city were transformed from spaces belonging to children into spaces meant for adults and "accompanied children" (p. 287). While Karsten (2005) acknowledges that contemporary societies offer new activities and possibilities for children's play, she argues that the "supervised culture" (p. 289) of childhood and children's play today is increasingly "focused in terms of time, space and activity" (p. 289). The diversity of play, and the space and time children have to play outdoors, thus appears to have diminished greatly. Rasmussen (2004) similarly examined the tendency for contemporary children in Denmark, as opposed to three decades ago, to be mainly confined to playing within three settings: the home, the school and institutions, and finally, facilities designated for children's recreation. She finds that these specific "places for children", created by adults and designated for children's use differ from what she calls "children's places", which represent how children create and relate to places that are not officially designated to them, and which are sometimes not meant for children's play. These two kinds of places are not mutually exclusive; children also create places for themselves within those that have been designated for them, climbing trees in a school playground, for instance, an activity that was normally forbidden (Rasmussen, 2004). However, the increasing confinement of places designated for children's play – "places for children" – and the tendency toward a greater regulation of time and space for children's activities, has meant that although "free" time and play are lauded and encouraged, the play predominantly engaged in these places cannot be considered to be free. As Rasmussen (2004) writes, "when 'free time' is spent in an institutional context, it is not experienced as quite free" (p. 169).

As such, in the 19th and early 20th centuries children's play underwent numerous transformations: self-directed games and play activities (that will be later defined as "free play") became increasingly directed towards specific goals (e.g., education, fitness) and involved organised games in designated places. The focus on individual satisfaction and personal reward through play was also replaced by group rewards, including public recognition through team sports and trophies. These transformations were evident in many industrialised countries by the early 20th century. For instance, Reiger (1985) writes of play in early 20th-century Australia:

> "children in busy cities" no longer knew how to play with freedom and naturalness, but organized games were referred to as training for "the game of life" in which challenge and competition were seen as important.
>
> (p. 170)

What this research and these play transformations demonstrate is that contemporary concerns about children's play are not new. Already in the late 19th and early 20th centuries, the search for techniques to control, standardise and institutionalise play became increasingly structured through the application of science to children's play and the desire for play to serve a concrete purpose (Frost, 2010). Referring to Johan Huizinga an eminent play theorist whose book *Homo Ludens* (1938) provides an historical and cultural analysis of the development of mostly western and European civilisation through what he calls the "play element", Malaby (2009) argues that Huizinga already

> felt that the play-element had been on the wane in Western civilization since the eighteenth century, threatened by the drive for efficiency and the routinization of experience it brought.
>
> (p. 210)

As such, underlying the trends towards increasingly structured, routinised and organised play is quite a long history of pushing for efficiency in play experiences, all with the possibility of greater productivity.

Contemporary perspectives: "free play", but still a means to an end

Beginning in the late 20th century there was a steep increase in research on play particularly in the field of education, and especially since the year 2000 (Cheng & Johnson, 2010). For instance, much of the contemporary research around play has come from the fields of child education and psychology. This research has examined how pretend play, role-playing and dramatic play advance children's psychological and academic development (Santer et al., 2007; Lillard, Lerner et al., 2013), has shown how playing with patterns and shapes and enumerating objects "supports the burgeoning mathematician" (p. 3), or has emphasised the critical importance of physical play for the development of the brain's frontal lobes (Hirsh-Pasek & Golinkoff, 2008). As such, in continuity with historical work, contemporary research on play re-emphasises – and assumes – that play is a critical means for optimal childhood educational and psychological development and that it is a way to promote, and further advance, certain qualities in children for later life.

Although much of this play research is based on the premise that children's play is "free", contemporary advocates of "free" play frequently suggest that play was freer, less confined, less institutional in the past, and there is a prominent debate and growing discussion about what is meant by play that is defined as "free". Santer et al. (2007) have conducted a literature review of research on free play in childhood and they define it as:

> children choosing what they want to do, how they want to do it and when to stop and try something else. Free play has no external goals set by adults and has no adult imposed curriculum. Although adults usually provide the space and resources for free play and might be involved, the child takes the lead and the adults respond to cues from the child.
>
> (p. xi)

However, paradoxically, while play – and free play – are valued and praised as important, in some settings play is also attributed the reputation of being frivolous and unnecessary. Sutton-Smith (1995) argued in the mid-1990s that:

> strangely, it is quite easy to find educators and administrators and politicians who act in a practical way as if play is of no damn use whatsoever by closing playgrounds, by abolishing recess and by organizing children's free time in every possible way.
>
> (p. 279)

These claims are substantiated by more recent trends in some American school settings where play is being eliminated from the curriculum in place of academic learning (Cheng & Johnson, 2010; Elkind, 2007; Fisher, Hirsh-Pasek, Golinkoff, & Gryfe, 2008; Hewes, 2009;

Hirsh-Pasek & Golinkoff, 2008). Yet, Sutton-Smith (1995) also argues that:

> since the death of Puritanism it has not been easy to find a self-respecting scholar of childhood who would announce that play is of no damn use whatsoever.
>
> (p. 279)

As such, while the specific place for play may be debated within the education system in North America, most researchers of childhood play agree that diverse forms of play – and free play – are a means of advancing children's healthy and optimal development (della rosa, 2011; Elkind, 2007; Hirsh-Pasek & Golinkoff, 2008; Lytle, 2003; Roskos & Christie, 2001, 2007; Youell, 2008).

Furthermore, it is also evident in these discussions that although the ideal-type of play is defined as free and unstructured, playing is still most often promoted as a means to achieve something else, to gain some kind of benefit. Cohen (1993) has argued that this tension between the intrinsic value of play as free and unstructured and the desire to regulate, confine and control children's play for specific purposes (a tension which already emerged in the 19th century) has remained strong in contemporary psychological play research:

> Today, few psychologists would argue against play or fantasy but the feeling still persists that such frivolous activities need to be justified by being in the service of reality. The right games should spur the best development.
>
> (Cohen, 1993, p. 13)

Lester and Russell (2014) call this the "'deferred benefits' approach" (p. 246) to play, where playing "serves something outside of playing" (p. 246). They argue that child development is viewed as a kind of maturation process, in which a child is "achieving full potential" for what it needs to become a good, and healthy adult. They write:

> Play can be commandeered to support this progression thereby assuming an instrumental value that promotes desirable play behaviors – those that clearly contribute to growing up – while at the same time censuring apparently purposeless, trivial and other undesirable play forms.
>
> (p. 245)

As such, contemporary discussions of play also present a paradox, one in which a desire to value-free, spontaneous and unstructured play for children is linked to the underlying value that play should also serve a productive purpose. With this in mind, the next section discusses the widespread rhetoric of play as a means for promoting children's progress.

The rhetoric of "play as progress" and fostering productive citizens

The discussions about how play can be conceptualised and studied was central to the work of the prolific play theorist, Brian Sutton-Smith. Sutton-Smith examined the controversies around play, in his book entitled *The Ambiguity of Play* (1997). In this book Sutton-Smith argues that play is virtually inaccessible as an object for scientific and social scientific study mostly due to the ambiguities that are inherent to it. These ambiguities, he suggests, result from rhetorical underpinnings or systems of value in academic disciplines and which result in distinct disciplinary perspectives on what play is, how it is studied, and how it is analysed and promoted (Sutton-Smith, 1997). Sutton-Smith (1997) discusses seven rhetorics (i.e., disciplinary narratives and ideological values) underlying different approaches to play (p. 8). He discusses four traditional rhetorics of play (of fate, of power, of identity and of frivolity), and three modern rhetorics (of progress, of the imaginary and of the self).

Of particular relevance is what Sutton-Smith (1997) has identified as the dominant rhetoric of "play as progress" which holds that "children . . . adapt and develop through their play" (p. 9). He argues that this rhetoric is currently dominant in western industrialised countries and that it has a strong influence on how play is currently perceived and studied (Sutton-Smith, 1997). As evidenced by some of the literature presented earlier in this chapter, Sutton-Smith (1997) has also observed that, since the late 18th and early 19th centuries, educators in particular have viewed play and playfulness as critical components of children's moral, social, psychological and cognitive development. Since then, according to Sutton-Smith (1997), play has been primarily valued as a means for child development and less for pleasure and enjoyment. He argues that especially because the 20th-century notions of progress and scientific rationality are so pervasive, the other six rhetorics of play have been marginalised; play that does not fit into the dominant rhetoric of "progress" is denigrated as frivolity (Sutton-Smith, 1997).

Some of the recent debates within psychology about whether (or not) the psychological benefits of play are in fact incontrovertible alludes to the possibility that this unwavering belief in play as crucial for children is influenced by Sutton-Smith's "rhetoric of play as progress" (Lillard, Lerner et al., 2013; Sutton-Smith, 1997; Lillard, Hopkins et al., 2013; Walker & Gopnik, 2013; Weisberg, Hirsh-Pasek, & Golinkoff, 2013). Indeed, both the psychological and education research on play discussed previously provide good examples of the disciplinary narrative of "play as progress". In this regard, as Cohen (2006) suggests, there is a long tradition, especially in the field of psychology, of viewing play as a means of learning something useful:

> while play may appear frivolous, it has to have a proper, serious explanation. It cannot just be; it has to have a purpose.
> (Cohen, 1993, p. 5)

We argue that the many attempts to justify the promotion of play by showing it is a useful tool for education, cognition or physical well-being may lead to a further instrumentalisation of play for children, one in which play becomes an obligation or begins to resemble work (we elaborate on this in Chapter 3). It is this observation – that play is increasingly instrumentalised – that is critical here. Play as an instrument to meet various ends speaks to what seems like a general societal desire for social practices and leisure activities to be productive – to contribute to progress and development. Currently, this desire for productivity, progress and development attaches itself readily to the social and leisure activities of children.

Producing and governing productive and "healthy" citizens

In the 19th and mid-20th centuries, during which there were enormous developments in scientific research, public hygiene, industrialisation, as well as two World Wars, a new social and political zeitgeist also emerged, particularly in the United States and western Europe, which greatly influenced how children's roles in society were perceived and the leisure activities they were encouraged to engage with (Foucault, 1980; Nadesan, 2010; Rose, 1999; Turmel, 2008; Chudacoff, 2007). As mentioned earlier in this chapter, by the early 20th century, a large body of knowledge about childhood brought with it a growth in social technologies of child regulation and the desire to establish authoritative measures to evaluate normal and healthy growth in childhood (Turmel, 2008). Children's social and leisure activities began to be promoted not only as a means to contribute to childhood cognitive and social development, but other qualities began to be increasingly promoted through children's playing as well, including optimal physical health and future economic productivity. The wish to promote these qualities through intervention on childhood activities thus developed alongside ideas about what constituted, and how to promote, a "normal" childhood (Turmel, 2008; Nadesan, 2010).

The growing focus on childhood normalisation at the time developed into what Nadesan (2010) calls a series of contemporary "formalized regimes of child discipline and character development" (p. 28). Linking this to the state's desire for productive (and healthy) citizens, Nadesan (2010) suggests that it was especially the growth of neo-liberal market rationalities that shaped domestic life and came to define prevalent attitudes towards children and child-rearing (Nadesan, 2010). Nadesan (2008) writes that families were made responsible for their child's exposure to numerous social and health risks (i.e., inactivity and overweight) for future illness (i.e., diabetes) in order to minimise the resulting social and economic costs. She writes:

> Today, vigilance is demanded of family-practice doctors, schoolteachers, and parents, all of whom are required to monitor children . . . for susceptibility to environmental dangers posed by "fat," lack of exercise, diet, television consumption, drugs, cigarettes, and so on. . . . [T]hese threats are believed to derive from lifestyle choices. . . . The costs of these "social contagions" are taken up within an economic calculus that includes health care, mental-health care (e.g., for depression), lost wages, disability costs, and the nation's long-term economic productivity.
>
> (p. 110)

It is thus, as of the late 20th to early 21st centuries, that children have been increasingly governed to be productive and healthy through what Nadesan (2010) calls an "invisible pedagogy", a pedagogy that appears to have increasingly integrated children's leisure as a key component for regulation. While this form of governing does not adopt the forceful authoritarianism of the past it employs "a panopticon of invisible pedagogies aimed at producing the subjects of liberal democracy" (Nadesan, 2008, p. 51). This can be likened to the notion of "biopedagogy", which has been theorised in the context of critical analyses of anti-obesity campaigns (Harwood, 2009). As we alluded to in Chapter 1, the concept of biopedagogy brings together Foucault's concept of biopower and the idea of pedagogy as a "pedagogy of bios". Biopedagogies aim to teach people – in this case children and their parents – about how to live, eat and generally how to behave in healthy and good ways (Harwood, 2009, p. 15). Analysing biopedagogies means questioning who the authorities (i.e., pedagogues) are who impart these instructions, and what the specific instructions are (i.e., discourses about what is true or good) that are being given. Such analyses thus question the strategies for intervention that ensure that individuals become "objects to be worked on, to be pedagogized" (Harwood, 2009, p. 24).

Biopedagogies also attend to modes of subjectification through which individuals are encouraged to work on themselves (Rabinow & Rose, 2006). Similar to the "invisible pedagogies" that aim to produce particular liberal subjects (Nadesan, 2008), biopedagogies – linked to the state's health and economic agenda – function not only at the level of the material body (i.e., to shape children's bodies), but also aim to produce particular (physically active and healthy) subjects. In the case of our work, these biopedagogies produce particular kinds of parents and children, who are taught about and come to adopt particular beliefs about their social, leisure and health practices (Burrows, 2009). We consider the discussions framing and promoting children's play and leisure activities as critical for progress and development to be part of a series of biopedagogies influencing children's physical health and social lives. Indeed, growing numbers of child health and development institutions and government agencies produce campaigns and information pamphlets informing the public about how much, and in which ways, children ought to play, be active, engage in recreation and leisure activities (see Chapter 3). These messages thus not only shape children's bodies, but also how children and families think about their leisure lives.

In other historical research, children's play spaces have been examined for how they promote a particular child subject as a way to secure a desired future citizenry. For instance, Kozlovksy (2008) analysed the development of adventure playgrounds built as part of the post–Second World War welfare state in Denmark and England. These "junk" playgrounds had the aim of reconstructing society through an investment in children and their play, and in their capacity as future citizens (Kozlovksy, 2008). Kozlovksy argued that unlike traditional playgrounds with fixed play structures that afforded a sort of external control over children's play activities, adventure playgrounds promoted experimentation in order to mobilise the child's internal inclination for play. The adventure playground was meant to induce in children the feeling of wanting to be free. Kozlovksy writes:

> in the case of the playground, power does not operate by dominating or disciplining subjects who were previously free, but rather by activating subjects and making them aspire to be free.
>
> (p. 172)

The healthy playing subject discussed in this book, and produced by public health discourses, clearly differs from Kozlovksy's (2008) description of a post-war subjectivity involving the ideals of freedom and engaged and empowered citizenry. What is in common, however, is the way play – and the possibilities made available for playing – have become a means to construct a particular child subject, who will contribute to a desired future society and to particular national goals. The next chapter picks up on this with a discussion of how institutions of public health in Canada have concretely taken up children's play in their physical activity interventions and promoted playing as a health practice in anti-obesity efforts. This ultimately reframes play as a form of physical activity, one that children are encouraged to enjoy, but which will importantly support a national agenda of combating childhood obesity.

References

Baker, B. M. (2001). *In perpetual motion: Theories of power, educational history and the child*. New York, NY: Peter Lang Publishing.

Boekhoven, B. (2009). *"Caution! Kids at Play?" Unstructured time use among children and adolescents*. Ottawa, Canada: The Vanier Institute of the Family.

Burrows, L. (2009). Pedagogizing families through obesity discourse. In J. Wright & V. Harwood (Eds.), *Biopolitics and the 'Obesity Epidemic': Governing bodies*. New York, NY: Routledge.

Cheng, M.-F., & Johnson, J. E. (2010). Research on children's play: Analysis of developmental and early education journals from 2005 to 2007. *Early Childhood Education Journal, 37*, 249–259.

Chudacoff, H. P. (2007). *Children at play: An American history*. New York, NY: New York University Press.

Cohen, D. (1993). *The development of play* (2nd ed.). London: Routledge.

Cohen, D. (2006). *The development of play* (3rd ed.). New York, NY: Routledge.

Della Rosa, E. (2011). The creative role of playfulness in development (Vol. 14). *Infant Observation, 14*(2), 203–217.

Elkind, D. (2007). *The power of play: How spontaneous, imaginative activities lead to happier, healthier children*. Berkeley, CA: Da Capo Press.

Fisher, K. R., Hirsh-Pasek, K., Golinkoff, R. M., & Gryfe, S. G. (2008). Conceptual split? Parents' and experts' perceptions of play in the 21st century. *Journal of Applied Developmental Psychology, 29*, 305–316.

Foucault, M. (1980). The politics of health in the eighteenth century. In C. Gordon (Ed.), *Power/knowledge: Selected interviews and other writings 1972–1977*. New York, NY: Pantheon Books.

Fröbel, F. (1887). *The education of man* (W. N. Hailmann, Trans.). New York, NY: D. Appleton and Co.

Frost, J. L. (2010). *A history of children's play and play environments: Toward a contemporary child-saving movement*. New York, NY: Routledge.

Gutman, M., & de Coninck-Smith, N. (2008). *Designing modern childhoods: History, space, and the material culture of children*. New Brunswick: Rutgers University Press.

Hart, R. (2002). Containing children: Some lessons on planning for play from New York City. *Environment and Urbanization, 14*(2), 135–148. doi:10.1177/09562478020140021l

Harwood, V. (2009). Theorizing biopedagogies. In J. Wright & V. Harwood (Eds.), *Biopolitics and the 'Obesity Epidemic': Governing bodies* (pp. 15–30). New York, NY: Routledge.

Hewes, J. (2009). *Let the children play: Nature's answer to early learning*. Montréal, Québec: Canadian Council on Learning, Early Childhood Learning Knowledge Centre.

Hirsh-Pasek, C., & Golinkoff, R. M. (2008). Why play = learning. In R. E. Tremblay, R. D. Peters & M. Boivin (Eds.), *Encyclopedia on early childhood development* (pp. 1–7). Montreal: Centre of Excellence for Early Childhood Development.

Huizinga, J. (1938/1949). *Homo Ludens: A study of the play-element in culture*. London: Routledge & Kegan.

Karsten, L. (2005). It all used to be better? Different generations on continuity and change in urban children's daily use of space. *Children's Geographies, 3*(3), 275–290.

Kozlovsky, R. (2008). Adventure playgrounds and postwar reconstruction. In M. Gutman & N. de Coninck-Smith (Eds.), *Designing modern childhoods: History, space, and the material culture of children*. New Brunswick: Rutgers University Press.

Lester, S., & Russell, W. (2014). Turning the world upside down: Playing as the deliberate creation of uncertainty. *Children, 1*, 241–260. doi:10.3390/children1020241

Lillard, A. S., Hopkins, E. J., Dore, R. A., Palmquist, C. M., Lerner, M. D., & Smith, E. D. (2013). Concepts and theories, methods and reasons: Why do the children (pretend) play? Reply to Weisberg, Hirsh-Pasek, and Golinkoff (2013); Bergen (2013); and Walker and Gopnik (2013). *Psychological Bulletin, 139*(1), 49–52.

Lillard, A. S., Lerner, M. D., Hopkins, E. J., Dore, R. A., Smith, E. D., & Palmquist, C. M. (2013). The impact of pretend play on children's development: A review of the evidence. *Psychological Bulletin, 139*(1), 1–34.

Lupton, D. (1995). *The imperative of health: Public health and the regulated body*. London: Sage Publications.

Lytle, D. E. (2003). *Play and educational theory and practice* (Vol. 5). Westport, CT: Praeger Publishers.

Malaby, T. M. (2009). Anthropology and play: The contours of playful experience. *New Literary History, 40*, 205–218.

Nadesan, M. (2008). *Governmentality, biopower, and everyday life*. New York, NY: Routledge.

Nadesan, M. (2010). *Governing childhood into the 21st century: Biopolitical technologies of childhood management and education*. New York, NY: Palgrave Macmillan.

Pellegrini, A. D. (1995). *The future of play theory: A multidisciplinary inquiry into the contributions of Brian Sutton-Smith*. Albany, NY: State University of New York Press.

Postman, N. (1994). *The disappearance of childhood*. New York, NY: Vintage Books Inc.

Rabinow, P., & Rose, N. (2006). Biopower today. *BioSocieties, 1*, 195–217.

Rasmussen, K. (2004). Places for children – Children's places. *Childhood, 11*, 155–173.
Read, J. (2006). Free play with Froebel: Use and abuse of progressive pedagogy in London's Infant Schools, 1870-c.1904. *Paedagogica Historica, 42*(3), 299–323.
Read, J. (2011). Gutter to garden: Historical discourses of risk in interventions in working class children's street play. *Children & Society, 25*(6), 421–434. doi: 10.1111/j.1099-0860.2010.00293.x
Reiger, K. M. (1985). *The disenchantment of the home: Modernizing the Australian family*. Melbourne: Oxford University Press.
Rivkin, M. S. (1997). The schoolyard habitat movement: What it is and why children need it. *Early Childhood Education Journal, 25*(1), 61–66.
Rose, N. (1999). *Governing the soul: The shaping of the private self* (2nd ed.). London: Free Association Books.
Roskos, K. A., & Christie, J. F. (2001). Examining the play – Literacy interface: A critical review and future directions. *Journal of Early Childhood Literacy, 1*(1), 59–89.
Roskos, K. A., & Christie, J. F. (2007). Play in the context of the new preschool basic. In K. A. Roskos & J. F. Christie (Eds.), *Play and literacy in early childhood: Research from multiple perspectives* (2nd ed., pp. 83–100). New York, NY: Erlbaum.
Santer, J., Griffiths, C., & Goodall, D. (2007). *Free play in early childhood: A literature review* (I. Cole-Hamilton, Ed.). London: National Children's Bureau.
Smith, P. K., & Pellegrini, A. D. (2005). *The nature of play: Great apes and humans*. New York, NY: The Guilford Press.
Sutton-Smith, B. (1995). Conclusion: The persuasive rhetorics of play. In A. D. Pellegrini (Ed.), *The future of play theory: A multidisciplinary inquiry into the contributions of Brian Sutton-Smith* (pp. 275–296). Albany, NY: State University of New York.
Sutton-Smith, B. (1997). *The ambiguity of play*. Boston, MA: Harvard University Press.
Turmel, A. (2008). *A historical sociology of childhood: Developmental thinking, categorization and graphic visualization*. New York, NY: Cambridge University Press.
Twain, M. (1917). *The adventures of Tom Sawyer*. New York, NY: Harper.
Walker, C. M., & Gopnik, A. (2013). Pretense and possibility – A theoretical proposal about the effects of pretend play on development: Comment on Lillard et al. (2013). *Psychological Bulletin, 138*(1), 40–44.
Weisberg, D. S., Hirsh-Pasek, K., & Golinkoff, R. M. (2013). Embracing complexity: Rethinking the relation between play and learning: Comment on Lillard et al. (2013). *Psychological Bulletin, 139*(1), 35–39.
Youell, B. (2008). The importance of play and playfulness. *European Journal of Psychotherapy and Counselling, 10*(2), 121–129.

Chapter 3

Active play
When playing becomes a job

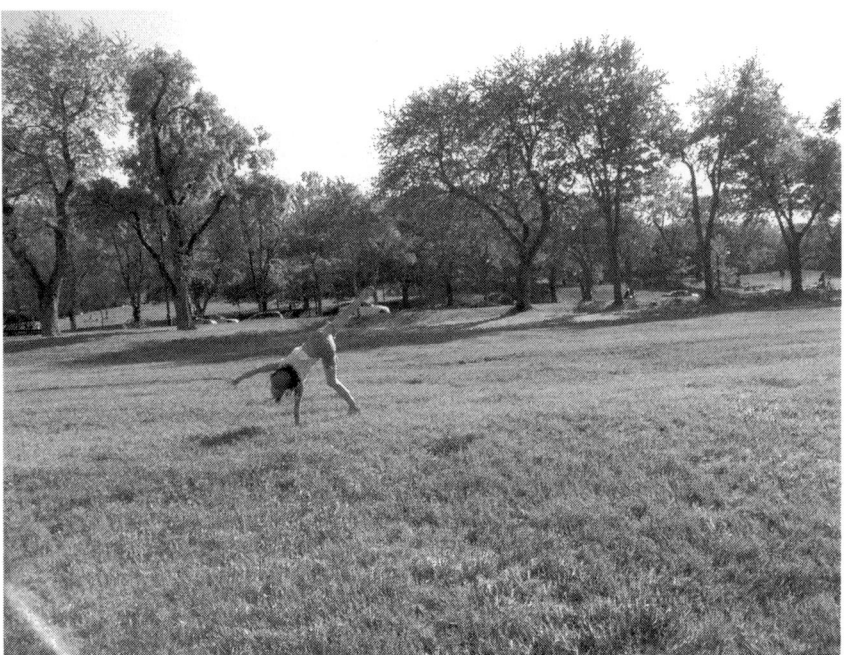

Figure 3.1 Charlotte (8 years old) wanted to be photographed doing a cartwheel.

Introduction

On May 27, 2011, *Le Soleil*, a Québec city (Canada) daily newspaper, published an article with the title "Kids' Gym in Quebec". The article, partly promotional, was announcing the June opening of the first Quebec "Petit Gym", a gym entirely dedicated to children between the ages of 4 months to 12 years of age. While the "Little Gym" concept is not new (in fact, it originated in 1976 under the auspices of kinesiologist

Robin Wes, *The Little Gym*, 2018), the idea of gyms for children is a useful entrée into the idea that children's play has rapidly become an activity that has a health aim, and one that requires effort or work. In this sense, play-time appears to have become an opportunity for children to work-out, the very raison-d'être for these new gyms. While not specifically focusing on the "Little Gym" concept, this chapter will explore the ways in which public health and physical activity promotion organisations may be contributing to changes in how children's play is conceived as having a very specific purpose of health improvement.

The contemporary public health interest in children's play appears to be informed by converging areas of research on children's play (Chapter 2) as well as by fears that there are decreasing opportunities for children to play and that changing leisure activities may have negative consequences for children's physical health. In this chapter, we discuss how growing concerns about children's physical health are redefining children's play, particularly the efforts to reduce childhood obesity. These concerns are mobilising innovative solutions for addressing children's inactivity levels, notably, children's leisure and play activities are becoming the new and increasingly popular targets of physical activity intervention. Through this, a broader health discourse is developing around children's play and its utility for addressing childhood obesity.

What makes the emerging public health discourse on play so pertinent for investigation is also what differentiates it from other disciplinary accounts of play (i.e., psychology and education, see Chapter 2). As a governmental institution, public health has an extensive reach, both influencing scientific research and having concrete societal application. It is thus distinct in its role of incorporating and regulating social practices as part of its health mandates. That is, numerous social activities indirectly related to health (i.e., walking or sitting, food consumption, sex) have been brought within the interest areas of public health authorities, who provide recommendations for the population about how often, and in which ways it is healthiest to, for example, walk, sit, eat or have sex.

The Public Health Agency of Canada (2003) defines the field of public health:

> Public health can be described as the science and art of promoting health, preventing disease, prolonging life and improving quality of life through the organized efforts of society. As such, public health combines sciences, skills, and beliefs directed to the maintenance and improvement of the health of all people through collective action.
> (PHAC, 2003, Chapter 3, p. 46)

Highlighting this definition is relevant as it not only explicitly underscores the value-based nature of public health practice as both a "science and art" whose practice depends on the "sciences, skills and beliefs", but it also emphasises the authority that public health wields when bringing together "organised efforts of society" and "collective action" for surveying and managing the health of the population. Specifically regarding the topic of children's play, a public health approach cannot be considered to have a value-free basis, and yet this particular approach has the potential to shape broad understandings of, and discourses on, children's contemporary and future leisure activities. Understanding the underlying values and assumptions that shape the public health interventions on children's play are thus critical. Before addressing the values and assumptions inherent in public health interventions on play, in the next section we discuss some of the contexts that have led to the emergence of the public health interest in children's leisure activities, and outline the ways in which it addresses children's play.

Public health, childhood obesity and the development of "active play"

Obesity epidemic and physical activity guidelines

The specific interest of public health institutions in contemporary children's leisure activities has developed within the context of increasing concerns about the growing rates of childhood obesity. Since the mid-1990s, according to public health officials, one of the most significant health issues to be addressed by public health in Canada is childhood obesity (Fox, 2004; Gard, 2010; Gard & Wright, 2005; McLaren, Zarrabi, Dutton, Auld, & Emery, 2012; Rich, Monaghan, & Aphramor, 2010; Shields, 2006; Stephen, 2006; Whitlock, Williams, Gold, Smith, & Shipman, 2005; WHO, 2010a; Wright & Harwood, 2009). Indeed, obesity in childhood has become a topic of significant concern globally with prevalence measures suggesting that rates of childhood obesity and overweight are steadily climbing in countries around the world, while physical activity levels for children are decreasing worldwide (WHO, 2000). All of this has prompted suggestions that obesity levels amongst children have reached epidemic proportions (Janssen et al., 2005; Shields, 2006; Stephen, 2006; WHO, 2010a).

In Canada, as in the United States and in a growing number of European and African countries (Ebbeling, Pawlak, & Ludwig, 2002; Onywera et al., 2013; Tremblay et al., 2014), there has been a surge of interest in measuring, evaluating and taking action on physical inactivity and obesity in the population, particularly among children and youth (PHAC, 2010; WHO, 2004; WHO, 2010b; WHO, 2012a; Kohl et al., 2012; Piggin & Bairner, 2016; WHO, 2010a). In terms of global numbers, the WHO (2012a) suggests that in 2012 there were an estimated 170 million children and youth (those under the age of 18) considered to be overweight. In Canada, an expert panel created for the *Obesity Canada Clinical Practice Guidelines* found that, in 2004, 26% of Canadian children and adolescents between the ages of 2 and 17 were overweight and that the rate of obesity had increased over the previous 15 years to 10% among boys and 9% among girls (Lau et al., 2007). According to the report Parliament of Canada's *Healthy Weights for Healthy Kids Report* (Parliament of Canada, 2007), Canada's rate of childhood obesity in 2007 ranked fifth out of 34 countries making up the *Organisation for Economic Co-operation and Development (OECD)*. The report suggests that an important reason for increases in childhood obesity was that "only 49% are active during their leisure time, accumulating the equivalent of about one hour of walking a day" (p. 3). The report states:

> most Canadian children do not participate in the 90 minutes per day of moderate activity (e.g., walking) or vigorous activity (e.g., running, climbing, swimming), as recommended by Canada's Physical Activity Guides for Children and Youth.
>
> (p. 3)

Canadian public health institutions have thus become increasingly concerned about the consequences that might result from increasing childhood inactivity and obesity (Fogel, Miltenberger, Graves, & Koehler, 2010; McLaren et al., 2012; Stephen, 2006; WHO, 2012a; Parliament of Canada, 2007). For instance, in 2007, with the publication of the *Healthy Weights for Healthy Kids* (Parliament of Canada, 2007) report, the Government of Canada decided to focus increased attention on childhood obesity prevention and allocated new funds specifically to re-establish the organisation ParticipACTION[1] with the specific mandate of creating public awareness campaigns to combat the growing childhood obesity crisis in Canada (Tremblay, Kho, Tricco, & Duggan, 2010; Parliament of Canada, 2007). One of ParticipACTION's main partners was Active Healthy Kids Canada (hereafter, AHKC), a not-for-profit organisation established in 1994 to promote physical activity to children and youth through the provision of "expertise and direction to policy makers and the public on how to increase, and effectively allocate resources and attention toward physical activity" (Colley, Brownrigg, & Tremblay, 2012, p. 321). Between 2005 and 2014 AHKC produced annual *Report Cards on Physical Activity for Children and Youth* (Active Healthy Kids Canada, 2013), which broadly assessed and reported on the situation of physical activity among Canadian children and youth (Active Healthy Kids Canada, 2014).

In a combined effort between the *Canadian Society for Exercise Physiology (CSEP)* and the *Public Health Agency of Canada (PHAC)*, *Physical Activity Guidelines* were developed as a series of evidence-based recommendations outlining for Canadians how much physical activity they should engage in per day. Originally, the first *Guidelines* published in 1995 were developed for adults, and in 2002 a set of *Guidelines* was created for children (aged 6–9 years) and youth (aged 10–14 years). However, in 2011 the CSEP and PHAC released a second revised set of *Guidelines* for children and youth in an effort to more effectively promote physical activity using new evidence collected through working groups and expert consultations at both national and international levels (e.g., UK, USA, Canada, Australia) (CSEP, 2011a). These new *Guidelines* for youth aged 5 to 11 years were created to more accurately depict a "dose-response relationship between the volume of moderate- to vigorous-intensity physical activity and increased health benefits" and were based on evidence, which according to CSEP "shows that substantial health benefits can be achieved with physical activity in excess of 60 minutes per day" (CSEP, 2011a, p. 2). Most recently, in 2012 *Guidelines* were also created "for the early years, ages 0–4" (CSEP, 2012).

Considered the most up-to-date evidence on physical activity, the CSEP *Guidelines* have been widely disseminated by governmental and non-governmental organisations to inform interventions and advocacy around children's physical activity. Indeed, as a way to reach families and children directly, the *Guidelines* are complemented by creative workbooks for children and youth as "attractive age-specific 'magazines' with activity themes" (Sharratt & Hearst, 2007, p. S13). Similarly, parents, caregivers and teachers were offered resources "to assist them in their roles as intermediaries" (p. S13) in helping children and youth achieve the recommended levels of physical activity. For Canadian physical activity promoters, the CSEP *Physical Activity Guidelines* thus provide "evidence-based" measures for how much physical activity children should be engaged in per day. However, while this evidence base was critical for interventions, the question of *how* to encourage children to attain higher levels of physical activity became another concern.

Public health and children's changing play landscape

The Canadian public health interest in children's play emerged in the midst of this obesity "crisis" and in the context of the multi-disciplinary mobilisation around children's play. Indeed at around the same time (i.e., early 2000s) a growing number of researchers and play advocates were making critical observations about the changing nature of contemporary childhood. Concerns included "declines" in opportunities and time to play, the changing nature of leisure activities and, of course, the concurrent growing rates of childhood obesity. One main observation about children's changing play landscape was that, according to these researchers, children were spending too little time playing outdoors. Reductions in outdoor play were in part attributed to the popularity of screen-based leisure pursuits and new forms of technology, all of which occur indoors (and are sedentary) (Chudacoff, 2007; Gard & Wright, 2005; Kimbro, Brooks-Gunn, & McLanahan, 2011). As children's outdoor play has been equated with physical activity, the increases in indoor play were linked to the increasing obesity rates amongst children, and the promotion of outdoor play became of prime public health importance.

Children's changing material and leisure culture has also been analysed and discussed by childhood studies scholars. This research has examined how recent changes such as the growing consumer economy, the availability of mass-produced games and toys and the changing physical spaces for play are reshaping children's relationship to their leisure activities (Clarke, 2008; Ito, 2008). The continuing effects of modernisation and societal changes have specifically impacted children's outdoor leisure and play, since many outdoor spaces that were previously used for play were redeveloped and are no longer available for children (Chudacoff, 2007; Gutman & de Coninck-Smith, 2008). As Freund and Martin (2004) suggest:

> residential neighbourhoods used to have wild spaces and secret places in which children could develop psychomotor and social fitness through free play, apart from adults. Such health-supporting spaces and places are rendered too distant by "car-scale" or too unsafe by car traffic. The ways in which our neighbourhoods are constructed, around car-culture, reduce the potential for play.
> (p. 276)

Furthermore, sedentary indoor leisure activities, especially those that are screen-based, also became the targets of new public health interventions

(Jakes et al., 2003; Gard & Wright, 2005). Although sedentary play includes any form of leisure activity that is not physically active, the kind of playing that received the most attention from public health was screen time (e.g., television, computers/tablets/phones, video games). The danger was seen to be its growing appeal and popularity and thus its propensity to detract from physically vigorous outdoor play (Bailey and McInnis, 2011; Adachi-Mejia et al., 2007; de Jong et al., 2013; Fogel et al., 2010; Marshall, Biddle, Gorely, Cameron, & Murdey, 2004; Thomson, Spence, Raine, & Laing, 2008). Chudacoff (2007) notes that already in the 1960s, television watching was deemed to be "destroying children's sense of values" and there was already the fear that television was beginning to replace "active healthy play with passive, sedentary apathy" (Chudacoff, 2007, p. 166). As such, while general concerns about screen technologies and leisure are not new, they have intensified, and, over the last decade, Canadian public health institutions have actively discouraged sedentary screen-play. For instance, in parallel to their *Physical Activity Guidelines*, the CSEP has also created a series of *Sedentary Behaviour Guidelines* which present the maximum amount of time during which infants, children and youth should be sedentary or engaged in screen time (CSEP, 2011b, 2012).

As such, it is over the last two decades, amid discussions of a changing childhood and a looming (or already developed) obesity crisis, that children have become the objects of interventions aimed simultaneously at increasing the opportunities for children's play and at preventing childhood obesity (Grove, 2012; WHO, 2012b; Wyatt, Winters, & Dubberte, 2006). Specifically in the wake of broader calls to address childhood obesity on a global scale (WHO, 2000), public health organisations in countries such as the USA, Canada, Australia and the UK have become particularly interested in the potential of interventions that promote "active" forms of play to address both the declines in play and the decreasing rates of physical activity. For instance, in Canada, one innovative approach was to increase the amount of physical activity children engage in not only during sports events or dedicated exercise activities (i.e., gym class at school), but also to promote physical activity as part of children's leisure and play-time (Booth, 2000; Dehghan, Akhtar-Danesh, & Merchant, 2005; Janssen et al., 2005; McDermott, 2007; McGall, McGuigan, & Nottle, 2011; Mulvihill, Rivers, & Aggleton, 2000; Salmon et al., 2005; Wyatt et al., 2006). To this end, the integration of children's play activities into materials promoting physical activity began to take on growing importance as a way to address children's physical (in)activity as a new anti-obesity tool.

Concept of "active play"

Since children's play was simultaneously being discussed by growing numbers of educators, psychologists, play advocates, urban planners and the media – particularly the concern that free play was on the decline – the Canadian public health interest in physically active play aligned well with this overall aim to reclaim and bring back children's play. What has emerged specifically from the attempts to promote physically active leisure to children is the formation of the new concept of "active play" defined as a type of physical activity. It is a concept that, in the context of physical activity promotion in Canada, has also become a measurable indicator of children's physical activity. Holt, Lee, Millar, and Spence (2015) draw on the work of the Canadian organisation *Active Healthy Kids Canada* to define "active play" in their article as

> a specific type of physical activity play that refers to child-initiated spontaneous and voluntary activities that include bursts of moderate to vigorous physical activity and that metabolic activity is well above resting rate.
>
> (p. 1)

"Active play" is thus a concept in which ideas about freedom and spontaneity in play are merged with CSEP physical activity recommendations from their *Physical Activity Guidelines* (i.e., 30 minutes of moderate to vigorous physical activity per day). In this way, the promotion of active play includes the attempt to meld elements of the fun inherent in playing with the requirements of being physical fit.

The two main Canadian organisations have been engaged in examining and promoting children's physical activity – and active play – as part of their interventions are ParticipACTION and Active Healthy Kids Canada (AHKC). Both organisations widely promoted the CSEP recommendations for child and youth physical activity, endeavoured to mobilise government and non-government organisations for changes to the social and physical environments and aimed to influence family and peers, schools and communities to increase physical activity opportunities (Tremblay et al., 2015). Between 2005 and 2014, AHKC produced annual *Report Cards on Physical Activity for Children and Youth* which broadly assessed and reported on the state of physical activity among Canadian youth (AHKC, 2014). The evidence base for the *Report Cards* is compiled from various sources of research literature, expertise and government and non-governmental organisations in order to develop and evaluate indicators for physical activity related to different facets of children's lives (Colley et al., 2012, p. 321; ParticipACTION, 2015a; Tremblay et al., 2015). The indicators in the *Report Cards* are developed, refined and evaluated through consensus by a group of experts in physical activity research to assess children's activity levels in Canada and to evaluate the country's physical activity opportunities (AHKC, 2014).

According to an analysis of the impact of the AHKC *Report Cards*, *Impact of the Active Healthy Kids Canada Report Card: A 10-Year Analysis*, the authors write:

> the Report Card has achieved > 1 billion media impressions, distributed > 120,000 printed copies and > 200,000 electronic copies, and benefited from a collective ad value > $10 million. The Report Card has been replicated in 14 countries, 2 provinces, 1 state and 1 city. AHKC has received consistent positive feedback from stakeholders and end-users, who reported that the Report Card has been used for public awareness/education campaigns and advocacy strategies, to strengthen partnerships, to inform research and program design, and to advance and adjust policies and strategies. Collectively, the evidence suggests that the Report Card has been successful at *powering the movement to get kids moving*, and in achieving demonstrable success on immediate and intermediate outcomes, although the long-term goal of improving the PA of Canadian children and youth remains to be realized.
>
> (Tremblay, Barnes, & Cowie Bonne, 2014, p. S3 190, emphasis in original)

It was in 2008 that the link between the declines in children's play (i.e., outdoor play) and childhood obesity was explicitly concretised in Canada through the integration and promotion of the concept of "active play" in physical activity interventions. Indeed, in their 2008 *Physical Activity Report Card for Children and Youth* (AHKC, 2008), AHKC included the new indicator of "active play" to their repertoire of indicators, viewing it as an important component of children's physical activity. The authors defined active play as having the "essential qualities of play in general (that is, fun, freely chosen, personally directed, spontaneous)", however, they emphasised that active play "differs in one important area: energy expenditure ... active play involves physical activity at energy costs well above resting levels" (AHKC, 2012, p. 23).

Active play was thus added to one of the central existing physical activity categories where it was positioned alongside "sports", "physical activity" and "screen time" as a new indicator for children's physical activity. The *Report Card* announces:

Active play was identified as an important new indicator for 2008 because of increased observations by concerned citizens that children and youth simply don't play outside as much as they used to. Active play is critical to the healthy development of our children and youth, but are we making sufficient effort to facilitate this in their lives? Some have started to question whether society has gone too far in regulating the lives of children away from the free play that previous generations enjoyed and arguably, took for granted.

(AHKC, 2008, p. 23)

By the time the 2012 *Report Card* was being written, the entire Report Card (entitled *Is Active Play Extinct?*) was dedicated to active play and especially to dealing with the fears of its decline (see Figure 3.2). As such, it was within the span of 4 years that the notion of "active play" developed from a concept into a fully recognised form of physical activity.

With the inclusion of the concept of "active play" in the *Report Cards*, children's physically active leisure thus came to be viewed as one of the central health indicators to be measured, evaluated and finally promoted as a crucially important form of physical activity (Alexander, Frohlich, & Fusco, 2014). With the new indicator of "active play" entering the vocabulary of the *Report Cards*, there was an increased need to further distinguish and evaluate the merit of different types of children's leisure – play that is "active" and therefore deemed healthy, and play that is "inactive" an deemed unhealthy.

In partnership with AHKC, ParticipACTION also produced a set of campaigns geared towards children and youth between the ages of 5 and 18 years. These physical activity campaigns emphasised the need for children and youth to engage in the scientifically established healthy "doses" of physical activity per day (i.e., the 30 minutes per day suggested by CSEP) (CSEP, 2011a), and this especially during leisure activities. Based on the emphasis on active play in the AHKC *Report Cards* (i.e., *Is active play extinct?* in 2012), ParticipACTION also launched a new public campaign entitled *Bring Back Play!* (2012), which similarly focused on promoting active play and "encouraging parents to increase their children's physical activity levels by bringing back the fun games and unstructured active play that used to be a part of every childhood". The campaign aired on television and was available online to warn Canadians that children's play was disappearing, and that collective efforts were needed to bring back play for children (i.e., physically active play) (ParticipACTION, 2012; ParticipACTION, 2015b). In the *Bring Back Play!* campaign, ParticipACTION writes

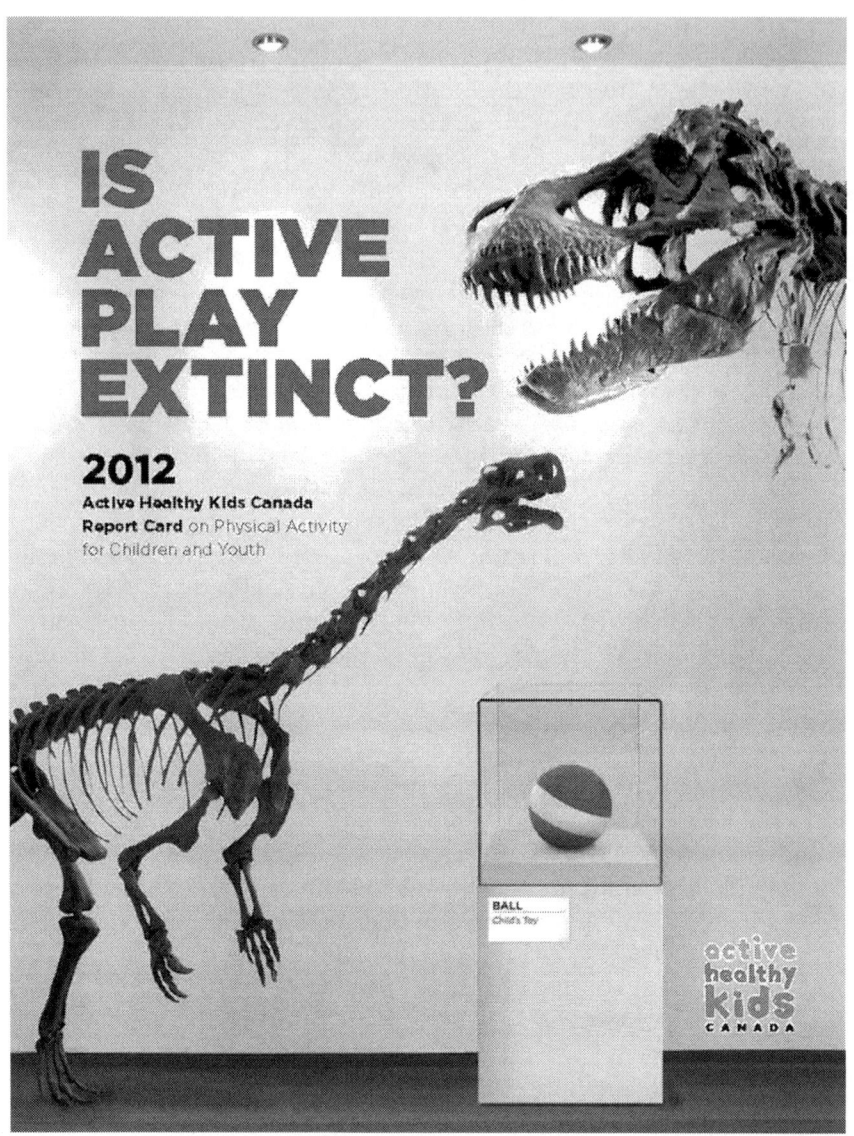

Figure 3.2 Front cover of the 2012 *Active Healthy Kids Canada Report Card*.

Note: Information from The Active Healthy Kids Canada 2012 Report Card on Physical Activity for Children and Youth has been provided with permission from Active Healthy Kids Canada. Active Healthy Kids Canada (2012). *Is Active Play Extinct? The Active Healthy Kids Canada 2012 Report Card on Physical Activity for Children and Youth*. Toronto: Active Healthy Kids Canada. A summary of the 2012 Report Card and the long-form version are available at www.activehealthykids.ca.

With only 5% of kids meeting the Canadian Physical Activity Guidelines of 60 minutes of physical activity EVERY day, play might be one of the easiest, most affordable and fun ways for our kids to get moving – if we all make the effort to Bring Back Play.
(ParticipACTION, 2012)

Since ParticipACTION's workbooks (mentioned earlier) and their televised and social media campaigns reach children and families directly (via television and the internet), they appear to be one important means through which the values of healthy active play are instilled in children's lives. Some of the workbooks are created to encourage children to learn to monitor, tabulate and evaluate their own active play. For instance, the workbook *Active Ways to Play!* (ParticipACTION, 2011a) encourages children to record their activities (provided they are active) and then gauge whether they are improving their physical activity levels each week:

Pick an activity that you love or try a new one. Don't forget to track how much time you spend doing your activity each week. See if you can beat your weekly total. Now turn off the TV and all your electronic toys and get ready, get set, PLAY!
(p. 2)

As such, ParticipACTION's campaigns further underscore that children's play is an area primed for physical activity intervention. Yet, what appears to be at the heart of these messages is that while it is assumed to be fun for children, active play should, first and foremost, involve the expenditure of energy so children can meet CSEP's *Physical Activity Guidelines*.

Another trend emerging from the overall concern about decreasing rates of physical activity and the rise of screen-play and electronic gaming – in the context of making physical activity fun – is the development of new technologies and electronic games that involve physical activity, termed "exergaming" (Bailey & McInnis, 2011; Barnett, Cerin, & Baranowski, 2011; Fogel et al., 2010; O'Loughlin, Dugas, Sabiston, & O'Loughlin, 2012; Shayne, Fogel, Miltenberger, & Koehler, 2012). For instance, Fogel et al. (2010) suggest that while video gaming is generally considered to be a factor contributing to childhood obesity, exergaming is a newer gaming technology, which reinforces physical activity in children. O'Loughlin et al. (2012) suggest that many adolescents exergame at intensities that would allow them to reach physical activity levels, such as those recommended by the CSEP's *Physical Activity Guidelines*. For some public health researchers, the promotion of exergaming therefore turns a vice into a virtue: advancing a new form of screen or electronic play to capitalise on children's enjoyment of video gaming while also addressing the public health of inactivity and childhood obesity.

However, despite the positive claims and the appeal of exergaming to increase children's physical activity, there have been critiques launched at the exergaming industry as well as the focus on fitness (and the related fitness equipment) more generally for children. For instance, some researchers have voiced reservations regarding the possible displacement of other kinds of physical activity (notably those that are outdoors) by exergames, and others have emphasised the potential adverse effects associated with active gaming, such as addiction or increased aggression (CFLRI, 2011; Daley, 2009). Some have also critiqued the way "crisis discourses" and an "alarmist rhetoric" (van der Schee & Boyles, 2010, p. 174) around childhood obesity are used as a strategy to justify and promote the use of commercial exergaming equipment in American schools (van der Schee & Boyles, 2010). These critiques are specifically aimed at the over-commercialisation of children's leisure activities.

It is through various attempts to intervene on children's obesity and physical activity levels then that public health and physical activity associations have become increasingly drawn to children's leisure activities and play-time, and specifically with reshaping it for the purposes of physical health. This is the angle our critique takes, and we continually ask whether this way of addressing children's leisure, through a public health and physical activity lens, may affect children's play – their understandings and possibilities for play – in unintended and possibly negative ways. We address this in the next section of this chapter.

Assumptions and values underlying the promotion of "active play"

Public health and play – a problematic combination?

As elucidated in the definition of public health at the outset of this chapter, public health is situated at the intersection of scientific knowledge and skills on the one hand, and of societal beliefs and values on the other, and, as such, public health discourses, directives and prescriptions addressing children's health hold significant influence over children's social and leisure experiences. Already in the late 20th century, the fragmenting of traditional expertise around childhood (i.e., teachers, paediatricians) and the emergence of new and varied sources of information about optimal child health and well-being (i.e., internet sites etc.) resulted in contemporary children being increasingly labelled, by public health authorities among others, as being "at risk" of various new afflictions such as "spending too much time in front of the computer, from obesity, from underachieving schools, and from environmental toxins" (Nadesan, 2010, p. 3).

This focus on governing the numerous risky facets of children's social and physical lives can also be seen as enduring in, and as expressed through, the new forms of governance of children's play within public health. While these efforts are ostensibly meant to benefit children's health, the integration of play into public health interventions transforms play into an activity that is laden with primarily health ends. We question here whether the continued focus on the physical health advantages of play above other aspects of playing (i.e., pleasure, freedom, independence) might marginalise some of these aspects, reshaping play and its pleasure for children.

As the literature in the previous chapter demonstrates, the instrumentalisation of play is not new. Play has long been studied and valued as critical for different facets of children's development. Writing about the instrumentalisation of play, Sutton-Smith (1995, 1997) has launched critiques at the overall tendency to view play as an exclusively useful activity that has children's learning and development as its main function; a tendency he has termed the "play as progress" orientation (discussed in Chapter 2) (Sutton-Smith, 1995). Sutton-Smith (1995) argues that what underlies the tendency to view play as productive may have its roots in the Enlightenment ideals of rational control and the view of humanity as capable of progress. These ideals inform the necessity for social practices and leisure activities to be productive – to contribute to progress – and thus, as we suggest, can attach themselves readily to children's leisure activities.

Yet, when play is ascribed a physical health goal, it is instrumentalised in yet another way. Contemporary institutions of public health are central in the instrumentalisation of numerous social practices for health purposes (see Chapter 4), but it is increasingly evident in the way health concerns are entering the realm of children's leisure; indeed, the justification for the promotion of play within public health interventions occurs on the basis of its (i.e., play's) health potential. While the health benefits of play for children are not contested, what concerns us here is that public health is an institution of modernity in which the ideals of scientific and humanistic progress and values of rationality, utilitarianism and productivity inhere (Crawford, 2006). Taken up within a state institution such as public health, playing not only becomes a health-focused practice, but it becomes an instrument to help fill a public health agenda regarding childhood obesity. What elements of pleasure, fun and spontaneity might remain within children's play?

Meyer and Schwartz (2000) have questioned the potential problems arising when social practices in general are viewed through a public health lens. They point out that as a result of an adherence to the ideals of a holistic view of health, the "new" public health (Baum, 2008) extends its reach into all areas of life and tends to absorb social practices as part of the health domain. With this, health and social issues have come to be viewed as inextricably linked. The authors argue that this becomes problematic when the health lens, through which social issues (in our case, children's play) are viewed, narrows the scope of what is taken into account when considering the "social" (Meyer & Schwartz, 2000). That is, viewing play primarily within a productive health optic narrows the scope of what play can signify (i.e., relevant only for health and development) and thus also what can be included within its scope (i.e., play as active, healthy). As we noted in Chapter 1 and wish to reiterate, this is a process that Meyer and Schwartz (2000) have called the "public healthification" (p. 1189) of the social, which they liken to the well-known concept of "healthism" (Crawford, 1980, 2006; Skrabanek, 1994). Indeed, Crawford's (1980) notion of "healthism" appears to underlie the public health discourse on many social practices, including play. Viewed as a super-value (Crawford, 1980, 2006) the concept of health itself provides a principal justification for, and a significant force behind, the reshaping of children's play as a productive element contributing to children's physical health.

This "public healthification" can be seen in the way active play is introduced in the AHKC *Report Card* precisely because it has come to be viewed as a way to promote physical health in children. In their media campaigns and workbooks, organisations such as AHKC and ParticipACTION repeat that children's play is not a frivolous activity and should be valued because it is endowed with the potential to foster children's physical health and development. Play and leisure in this context are understood and valued as productive health activities.

In this instance, one can ask whether "active play", although described and promoted as fun, is actually more akin to schoolwork for children. The forms of play mandated by public health – those prescribed to be healthy, active, monitored, tabulated and evaluated – indeed appear to take on the quality of work (i.e., schoolwork). For instance, in one workbook, a lower grade is attributed to the category of children having done "less than 60 minutes of activity per week" and is accompanied by the following text: "Holy Cow! Do you realize that you've basically done nothing all week?"

(ParticipACTION, 2013, p. 1). Here, leisure activities that are not also physically active (at best 60 minutes per day) are described as "doing nothing". Play is only valued if it productively contributes to physical activity, and in this way it appears to become an obligation engendering qualities decidedly different from activities that are spontaneous and more freely chosen by children. By asking children to record, appraise and reform their leisure time according to these health prescriptions, play indeed takes on some of the characteristics of work. As Russell (2013) suggests:

> If play is colonised exclusively within this understanding, it becomes objectified and loses its defining characteristics: it is no longer autotelic, nor is it a display of children's power over real-and-imagined worlds. Ultimately, robbed of emotion and meaning, play itself becomes alienating, becoming less like play and more like work.
> (p. 171)

Despite this assertion, however, Russell (2013) also suggests that children will not necessarily succumb to this and will also "find ways to disturb the adult ordering of space and time in order to create spaces for play within lived space" (p. 171).

Other critiques have been aimed at the way leisure and free time are organised around fitness-focused activities – what can be called the "fitness movement". For instance, Freund and Martin (2004) have suggested that the fitness movement has in effect eliminated the time and freedom people have for engaging in what they call "undisciplined activities" that are playful and "unorganised". They write:

> The time available for playful uses of the body, or for undisciplined activity, or for altered states of consciousness (other than the intensely attentive) has shrunk. It has been compressed into the tiny lacunae of "free time": time that is not saturated by production or consumption disciplines. This time squeeze is aggravated by car-hegemonic organisations of movement space, particularly their tendency to disperse and to sever activity sites, including fitness sites (public parks, footpaths and swimming pools as well as private gyms and health clubs).
> (p. 277)

While Freund and Martin (2004) critique the fitness movement in which adults are generally implicated, this "fitness focus" can be found in discussions of children's health and in the way children's leisure time and activities are organised for physical activity, as with the "Little Gym" concept mentioned at the outset of this chapter. We argue that this leaves very little room for the kind of unstructured, unplanned activities that children can engage in during free play-time.

Furthermore, children from diverse social backgrounds engage differently in play activities, which is due in part to inequalities in the material and environmental resources available to children, as well as to differences in the amounts of time families have to dedicate to recommended forms of active play. For example, Kimbro et al. (2011) conducted one study of socio-economic differences affecting children's play. The authors first examined whether television watching versus outdoor play were associated with children's body mass index (BMI), and then they examined the relationship between children's BMI and various neighbourhood characteristics (e.g., SES, type of home, physical disorder in the neighbourhood) (Kimbro et al., 2011). The authors found that, as predicted, the number of hours of outdoor play was associated with lower BMI, and that, generally, watching television was associated with higher BMI (Kimbro et al., 2011). However, what surprised the authors was that children who lived in public housing (lower SES) played outdoors for more hours than those living in higher SES neighbourhoods, but they also watched more hours of television (Kimbro et al., 2011). They hypothesise:

> children in lower class households have much more unstructured time than do those in middle-class households, reflecting class differences not just in resources but also in child-raising philosophies.
> (p. 674)

The public health promotion of active outdoor play in order to achieve the prescribed 30 (or 60) minutes of physical activity per day, as well as the simultaneous discouragement of all sedentary and screen-based play (e.g., TV, computers), may not take the social economic differences of children's lives into account, and may thus only reflect the social, temporal, spatial and financial circumstances – and possibilities – of some families and children.

Active play for national prosperity

As we mentioned in Chapter 2, the public health governance of children's leisure and social activities can be understood as a form of biopedagogy linked to the state's health and economic agenda (Foucault, 1980; Harwood, 2009). Foucault (1980) had already discussed the new medical and public health authorities of the 18th century which were created with the role of regulating the population's health as well as their economic productivity (Nadesan, 2010; Rose, 1999). At the time, this meant an expansion of the reach of medical institutions beyond the individual to all aspects of society, including the family and especially children (Foucault, 1980). The family became interrelated with national prosperity primarily since it was considered a prominent and central site for the production of a state's future citizens (Foucault, 1980; Nadesan, 2010).

Viewing public health interventions promoting "active play" for obesity prevention as a form of pedagogy of the body – or biopedagogy – means examining interventions and problematising the normalising and regulating practices that inform families about how to become good and healthy citizens through recommendations about how to play "properly". Furthermore, the social and economic consequences linked to children's obesity reinforce the importance and value of active play, and in this way directly link children's play to the social and economic concerns of a country's public healthcare system. Several striking examples of this are exemplified in Canada with the campaigns and documents produced by ParticipACTION and AHKC and in advertisements of a leading Canadian sports equipment store (Canadian Tire, 2018).

In the work of ParticipACTION specifically, there has been a long-standing idea that physical activity is a significant component and symbol of Canadian national identity. For instance, Lamb Drover (2014) has suggested that, already in the 1970s, ParticipACTION explicitly drew on and helped construct a Canadian physical activity identity. Citing a 1981 ParticipACTION booklet that explicitly promotes the mandate of "not just getting individuals fit, but of building a fit nation" (p. 297), Lamb Drover (2014) suggests that this marketing strategy instigated the Canadian population to "perform their patriotism through physical activity" (p. 297). After funding was reinstated in 2007, ParticipACTION resurfaced and labelled itself "Canada's premier physical activity brand" (ParticipACTION, 2015a) and promoted physical activity as a component of Canadian national identity. In their 2015 policy statement entitled: *Healthy, Prosperous, United: An active Canada is a better Canada* (ParticipACTION, 2015b), national identity is explicitly promoted through physical activity:

> From our local playgrounds to our inspiring high-performance athletes, sport and physical activity are vital to the cultural fabric of our nation.
>
> (p. 2)

National identity has also been invoked to promote and valorise certain ways of playing, notably sports, which the organisation defines as particularly Canadian. As part of ParticipACTION's (2013) *Bring Back Play!* campaign, ideas are proposed for bringing back Canadian winter play. Families are urged to play actively outdoors, even when it is cold, suggesting it is part of being "Canadian":

> Let's warm up to winter and embrace what being Canadian is all about. Help us Bring Back Winter Play by getting outside for at least 60 minutes of active fun each day.
> (ParticipACTION, 2013)

Additionally, the sports, home and hardware company, Canadian Tire (2018), has pursued the promotion of "active" play for children's physical health. Drawing on the developing momentum around active play in Canada, their slogan *We all play for Canada* (Canadian Tire, 2013) provides another example of how play and physical activity have been linked to a very specific and sports-oriented Canadian citizenship. In a popular 2013 TV advertisement, Canadian Tire makes a direct link between children's play, health and national prosperity. The advertisement is evocative, and the text[2] is read over orchestral music that builds in momentum during the 1-minute advertisement. Opening piano music accompanies nostalgic archival footage of children happily playing outdoors, the past indicated by sepia colours and 1970s fashions. However, the mood changes with the words "but have you noticed ... play doesn't come out to play as much anymore". The video darkens as it shows a dilapidated basketball court, abandoned swings and present-day listless children lying on couches playing video games and watching TV. With a rallying call to "bring back play", the music, anthem-like, gains in intensity and crescendos as the video highlights children playing with different kinds of sports equipment, the National Hockey League's iconic Stanley Cup, Canadian sports heroes and children (all wearing the Canadian Tire logo) playing soccer, baseball, out in the backyard, at a park and swimming pool. The closing scene shows three children running up a hill together carrying a large Canadian flag. As they fade into the horizon, the last words are spoken: *We all play for Canada*.

Through this specifically Canadian perspective, it appears that playing sports outdoors has become a symbol of being *truly* Canadian; a citizen who displays a physical hardiness and "outdoorsy" character, by playing actively outside despite the weather conditions. The aim appears to be to unite Canadians in a collective effort to engage all children in this kind of active play, for the sake of children's health, but fundamentally, for producing healthy (productive) citizenship for the sake of Canada as a "nation".

The governing of children and adults to be, or become, healthy, "good" Canadian citizens can be understood through the concept of producing "subject positions", which MacNeill and Rail (2010) describe in their work on Canadian youth as a series of "codes for individuals to know how to act, behave and perform in social practices" (p. 176). In their research study entitled *Canadian Youth Constructions of Health and Fitness*, the authors argue that through the subject positions available for youth, youth are interpolated by political and health efforts to "produce themselves as healthy citizens and contribute to the reduction of national medicare costs" (p. 178). Based on their findings, MacNeill and Rail (2010) suggest that Canadian schools and sports/fitness-oriented summer camps have become "key sites where Canadian youth receive lessons and directives about transforming their individual bio-selves into 'active healthy living' citizens" (p. 175). Indeed, the public health– and physical activity–oriented campaigns, interventions, workbooks and sports advertisements that we have analysed and which incite children to play more actively are precisely the kinds of sites that offer subject positions for children through recommendations for how to become a healthy, actively playing and fit Canadian child.

Children's perspectives on play

In contrast to the public health perspective in which play is valued and promoted for its health potential, we found that many of the children who participated in our study made distinctions between different forms of play. They discussed forms of play that were both active and inactive, and described engaging in play for a variety of different reasons. One central theme that emerged was that for some children there was a distinction between activities that were purposeless and self-directed and those that were adult-led or scheduled. Indeed, while children described organised activities such as being on a sports team or taking lessons as rewarding and fun, some children also described this kind of scheduled activity as an obligation. Sebastien, an 11-year-old boy who said he loved playing soccer and wanted to join a competitive team was not unequivocally enthusiastic about all aspects of this:

> I have a lot of time to play, but sometimes, the days when I'm tired, I'd like it if there was, like, no obligations. Say soccer training, sometimes I am just so tired that I really don't feel like doing it. But it's always an obligation for me. Each time I'm told

> "Sebastien, you have to go to the practice", so even if I really don't feel like it, I go.

The sense of obligation attributed to particular kinds of scheduled playing also appeared to affect some children's enjoyment of play. In particular, these children mentioned feeling exhausted by their organised play schedules and that they wanted to take a break from these activities in order to make time for other forms of less organised play. For instance, Michel a 9-year-old boy, talked about the sports and music lessons he was involved in over the past year:

> I did take diving lessons, but that stopped because I took other lessons. And speed skating, I did that during the winter . . . for now, there's just the piano lessons. Because otherwise, you can't really do, "OK let's go to speed skating, OK now let's go to diving lessons, OK now let's go to swimming, OK, let's go to piano . . .!" Then it would be too exhausting and I'll start to say "ah, no! Not swimming!" and "ah no! Not diving!"

Michel later said that although he likes to be on a team, he prefers to be the one deciding what and how to play:

> Well, I like playing freely, because you can do whatever you want . . . it's just that sometimes it annoys me when a coach always says "OK, do that now, do this, do that" . . . I prefer to go about it slowly and afterwards to do whatever I want, then it's me who chooses what I do and not the coach. There's no one telling me what to do, I am the one who decides. And I can do whatever I want.

Children's descriptions of play activities as being obligations or as exhausting, and their desire for more self-determined play, emerged in relation to forms of play that they described as adult-led or structured and organised. Although just a small sample of children's interview excerpts are presented here, our findings overall have led us to question whether the sense of obligation and exhaustion that is linked to scheduled and organised play may in fact undermine the pleasure children can gain from their everyday leisure activities. Sociologist Roger Caillois' (1961) argument, while not strictly addressing children's play, nonetheless comes to mind here. He argues that when rules for everyday life infiltrate the universe of play, pleasure may in turn become work-like, an obligation (Caillois, 1961). This observation provokes us to consider whether play is being re-shaped (as an obligation or as work) when it is organised and structured to have a productive health function within a public health discourse.

The distinction that some children made between different ways of playing resonates with MacDougall, Schiller, and Darbyshire's (2004) research conducted with children about play, physical activity and sport. They suggest that children have strong affective associations with different kinds of leisure activities. Playing was viewed as distinct for children and associated with child-centredness, whereas sport was associated with being organised by adults. Children's affective associations with play and sport were also qualitatively different than children's associations with physical activity and exercise, which seemed to carry less meaning for children overall (MacDougall et al., 2004).

Our research also shows that different forms of play appear to be affectively distinct for children. For instance, we found that activities that would be defined as inactive or sedentary and which would not be actively promoted within public health, such as knitting, reading, playing computer games and drawing, were discussed by some children as providing a sense of soothing, calm or comfort when they were not feeling well, rather than explicitly eliciting pleasure or fun. These forms of play, which were specifically less active, were affectively important for children who described themselves as wanting time to think or who said they were feeling a bit low or sad. Sebastien's previous description of his soccer training above contrasts markedly with the way he discusses his drawing:

> Drawing is also when I feel that I have to let my imagination out. What I like about drawing is that there are no limits, you can draw pretty much anything . . . and when I'm done my drawing, what I like is that, well, I'm relaxed. I drew something. I had fun. It lets me draw the things that I imagine in my mind . . . because I really have a lot of imagination.

Moreover, Florence, an 8-year-old girl, said that although she liked to play basketball and hockey, playing in calm, quiet ways felt good when she was sad or alone:

> Sometimes I'm more sad. Say, you don't feel very good sometimes, well, you can just play, and this feels good . . . I read more, and I do what relaxes me . . . like knitting, and books . . . it feels good to do it when you are all alone.

Feeling good, relaxing or drawing imaginatively were some descriptions of how engaging in forms of sedentary play was affectively important for children. Henri, a 9-year-old boy, also said that playing and having fun for him was actually associated with engaging in any activity that simply interested him. He talks about doing a puzzle as an example:

> Playing for me is having fun, something that is enjoyable. It's not necessarily funny, but it's something that interests me. The puzzle for example, why do I like that? Because it works your mind and I find it really fun.

In light of children's narratives, we argue that when playing is framed within public health as an activity that should be primarily physically active, or when playing is organised to fit a particular schedule – in short, when play becomes efficient, compartmentalised and productive – the free and spontaneous quality of some forms of play, and the calm and quiet they can afford, may become increasingly marginalised, or deemed too frivolous at a time when children's free time is to be used productively for health.

Examining similar play and physical activity campaigns in New Zealand, Burrows (2010) has examined young children's engagement with physical activity, health and leisure. She discusses how a long-running government physical activity campaign called *Push Play* (Sport New Zealand, 2013) has solicited increasingly numerous everyday leisure activities for physical activity promotion purposes. Similar to the Canadian campaigns (e.g., *Think Again* and *Bring Back Play*, ParticipACTION, 2011b, 2013), New Zealand's *Push Play* campaign promotes the message that "children need to 'push play' every day by engaging in at least 60 minutes of physical activity" (Burrows, 2010, p. 156). As an example of how elements of youth culture become reshaped in this campaign, Burrows (2010) describes how "krumping", a creative and free-flowing dance adopted primarily by Pasifika youth in New Zealand, has been drawn into the "push play" campaign, and away from the margins, as a way to recruit youth to adopt physical activity. Burrows (2010) argues that with the adoption of krumping into physical activity promotion discourses, "krumping as a 'cultural practice' in effect is diluted, re-envisaged as yet another way to push play every day" (p. 157). Burrows' research underscores our argument here that a possible (un)intended consequence of taking up and systematically re-directing children's play as part of physical activity campaigns potentially transforms and redirects play experiences into obligations and activities that are experienced as exhausting (Alexander, Frohlich, &

Fusco, 2012; Frohlich, Alexander, & Fusco, 2012). Indeed, attributing physical health goals to children's play in this way risks evacuating some of the distinct qualities of play that appear to also be important to children (i.e., free, unstructured, spontaneous, self-determined, calm, quiet or inactive).

Having discussed how growing concerns about children's physical health (i.e., obesity) align with concerns about the decline in children's free and outdoor play and how this has mobilised solutions involving active play, and the implications for reshaping ideas about, and experiences of, play for children, we turn to the way discourses of public health have intervened on pleasurable activities more broadly. In the next chapter, we discuss this with respect to how pleasure is experienced in relation to various health-related social practices. Analysed as a new form of morality, we discuss how pleasure is prescribed in very specific ways in relation to health practices, including children's "active play".

Notes

1 ParticipACTION is a Canadian non-profit organisation founded in the 1970s to promote physical activity to Canadians and though shut down in 2001, it was re-launched in 2007 and funded by the Public Health Agency of Canada (PHAC).
2 The advertisement states: "Through seasons that changed and smiles that didn't, no company has shared this nation's passion for play like Canadian Tire. But have you noticed? . . . Play doesn't come out to play as much anymore. As a company that cares deeply about families knowing half our kids aren't active matters . . . for a country without strong children cannot stay strong. So Canadian Tire is rallying this country's most influential partners to bring back play. . . . And with it, all the confidence, creativity and strength that serves to remind: We all play for Canada" (Canadian Tire, 2013, our emphasis).

References

Active Healthy Kids Canada. (2008). *The active healthy kids Canada report card on physical activity for children and youth*. Toronto, Canada: Active Healthy Kids Canada.

Active Healthy Kids Canada. (2012). *Is active play extinct? Report card on physical activity for children and youth*. Toronto, Canada: Active Healthy Kids Canada.

Active Healthy Kids Canada. (2013). *About us: Who we are*. Retrieved March 2013 from www.activehealthykids.ca/AboutUs.aspx

Active Healthy Kids Canada. (2014). *Is Canada in the running? How Canada stacks up against 14 other countries on physical activity for children and youth*. Toronto, Canada: Active Healthy Kids Canada.

Adachi-Mejia, A. M., Longacre, M. R., Gibson, J. J., Beach, M. L., Titus-Ernstoff, L. T., & Dalton, M. A. (2007). Children with a TV in their bedroom at higher risk for being overweight. *International Journal of Obesity*, 31(4), 644–651.

Alexander, S. A., Frohlich, K. L., & Fusco, C. (2012). Playing for health? Revisiting health promotion to examine the emerging public health position on children's play. *Health Promotion International*, 29(1), 155–164.

Alexander, S. A., Frohlich, K. L., & Fusco, C. (2014). 'Active play may be lots of fun . . . but it's certainly not frivolous': The emergence of active play as a health practice in Canadian public health. *Sociology of Health & Illness*, 36(8), 1188–1204.

Bailey, B. W., & McInnis, K. (2011). Energy cost of exergaming: A comparison of the energy cost of 6 forms of exergaming. *Archives of Pediatric Adolescent Medicine*, 165(7), 597–602.

Barnett, A., Cerin, E., & Baranowski, T. (2011). Active video games for youth: A systematic review. *Journal of Physical Activity and Health*, 8(5), 724–737.

Baum, F. (2008). *The new public health* (3rd ed.). Melbourne: Oxford University Press.

Booth, M. (2000). What proportion of Australian children are sufficiently active? *Medical Journal of Australia*, 173(Suppl. 7), S6–S7.

Burrows, L. (2010). Push play every day: New Zealand children's constructions of health and physical activity. In M. O'Sullivan & A. MacPhail (Eds.), *Young people's voices in physical education and youth sport* (pp. 145–162). New York, NY: Routledge.

Caillois, R. (1961). *Man, play, games* (M. Barash, Trans.). Urbana, IL: University of Illinois Press.

Canadian Tire. (2013). *We all play for Canada*. Retrieved from http://weallplayfor canada.ca/ and http://m.youtube.com/watch?v=UAaOiEvjcGM

Canadian Tire. (2018). *Canadian Tire*. Retrieved from www.canadiantire.ca/en.html

CFLRI, & ParticipACTION. (2011). The influence of after-school programs on children's physical activity levels. In *The research file*. Ottawa, Canada: Canadian Fitness Lifestyle Research Institute.

Chudacoff, H. P. (2007). *Children at play: An American history*. New York, NY: New York University Press.

Clarke, A. J. (2008). Coming of age in Suburbia: Gifting the consumer child. In M. Gutman & N. de Coninck-Smith (Eds.), *Designing modern childhoods: History, space, and the material culture of children*. New Brunswick: Rutgers University Press.

Colley, R. C., Brownrigg, M., & Tremblay, M. S. (2012). A model of knowledge translation in health: The active healthy kids Canada report card on physical activity for children and youth. *Health Promotion Practice*, 13(3), 320–330.

Crawford, R. (1980). Healthism and the medicalization of everyday life. *International Journal of Health Services*, 10(3), 365–388.

Crawford, R. (2006). Health as a meaningful social practice. *Health: An Interdisciplinary Journal for the Social Study of Health, Illness and Medicine*, 10(4), 401–420.

CSEP. (2011a). *Canadian physical activity guidelines: For children 5–11 years*. Canadian Society for Exercise Physiology.

CSEP. (2011b). *Canadian sedentary behaviour guidelines: For children 5–11 years*. Canadian Society for Exercise Physiology.

CSEP. (2012). *Canadian physical activity and sedentary behaviour guidelines for the early years (aged 0–4 years)*. Canadian Society for Exercise Physiology.

CSEP. (2018). *About the Canadian society for exercise physiology*. Retrieved May 2017 from www.csep.ca/english/View.asp?x=460

Daley, A. J. (2009). Can exergaming contribute to improving physical activity levels and health outcomes in children? *Pediatrics*, 124(2), 763–771.

Dehghan, M., Akhtar-Danesh, N., & Merchant, A. T. (2005). Childhood obesity, prevalence and prevention. *Nutrition Journal, 4*, 24–32.

de Jong, E., Visscher, T. L. S., HiraSing, R. A., Heymans, M. W., Seidell, J. C., & Renders, C. M. (2013). Association between TV viewing, computer use and overweight, determinants and competing activities of screen time in 4- to 13-year-old children. *International Journal of Obesity, 37*(1), 47–53.

Ebbeling, C. B., Pawlak, D. B., & Ludwig, D. S. (2002). Childhood obesity: Public-health crisis, common sense cure. [Research Support, Non-U.S. Gov't Research Support, U.S. Gov't, P.H.S. Review]. *Lancet, 360*(9331), 473–482. doi:10.1016/S0140-6736(02)09678-2

Fogel, V. A., Miltenberger, R. G., Graves, R., & Koehler, S. (2010). The effects of exergaming on physical activity among inactive children in a physical education classroom. *Journal of Applied Behavior Analysis, 43*(4), 591–600.

Foucault, M. (1980). The politics of health in the eighteenth century. In C. Gordon (Ed.), *Power/knowledge: Selected interviews and other writings 1972–1977*. New York, NY: Pantheon Books.

Fox, K. R. (2004). Childhood obesity and the role of physical activity. *The Journal of the Royal Society for the Promotion of Health, 124*(1), 34–39.

Freund, P., & Martin, G. (2004). Walking and motoring: Fitness and the social organisation of movement. *Sociology of Health & Illness, 26*(3), 273–286. doi:10.1111/j.1467-9566.2004.00390.x

Frohlich, K. L., Alexander, S. A., & Fusco, C. (2012). All work and no play? The nascent discourse on play in health research. *Social Theory & Health, 11*(1), 1–18.

Gard, M. (2010). Truth, belief and the cultural politics of obesity scholarship and public health policy. *Critical Public Health, 21*(1), 37–48.

Gard, M., & Wright, J. (2005). *The obesity epidemic: Science, morality and ideology*. New York, NY: Routledge.

Grove, J. (2012). Bringing back play: ParticipACTION's Kelly Murumets. *Active for Life Magazine*. Retrieved from http://activeforlife.ca/bringing-back-play-kelly-murumets/

Gutman, M., & de Coninck-Smith, N. (2008). *Designing modern childhoods: History, space, and the material culture of children*. New Brunswick: Rutgers University Press.

Harwood, V. (2009). Theorizing biopedagogies. In J. Wright & V. Harwood (Eds.), *Biopolitics and the 'Obesity Epidemic': Governing bodies* (pp. 15–30). New York, NY: Routledge.

Holt, N. L., Lee, H., Millar, C. A., & Spence, J. C. (2015). 'Eyes on where children play': A retrospective study of active free play. *Children's Geographies, 13*(1), 73–88. doi:10.1080/14733285.2013.828449

Ito, M. (2008). Migrating media: Anime media mixes and the childhood imagination. In M. Gutman & N. de Coninck-Smith (Eds.), *Designing modern childhoods: History, space, and the material culture of children*. New Brunswick: Rutgers University Press.

Jakes, R. W., Day, N. E., Khaw, K.-T., Luben, R., Oakes, S., Welch, A., . . . Wareham, N. J. (2003). Television viewing and low participation in vigorous recreation are independently associated with obesity and markers of cardiovascular disease risk: EPIC-Norfolk population-based study. *European Journal of Clinical Nutrition, 57*, 1089–1096.

Janssen, I., Katzmarzyk, P. T., Boyce, W. F., Vereecken, C., Mulvihill, C., Roberts, C., . . . Health Behaviour in School-Aged Children Obesity Working Group.

(2005). Comparison of overweight and obesity prevalence in school-aged youth from 34 countries and their relationships with physical activity and dietary patterns. *Obesity Reviews: An Official Journal of the International Association for the Study of Obesity*, 6(2), 123–132.

Kimbro, R. T., Brooks-Gunn, J., & McLanahan, S. (2011). Young children in urban areas: Links among neighborhood characteristics, weight status, outdoor play, and television watching. *Social Science & Medicine*, 72(5), 668–676.

Kohl, H. W. R., Craig, C. L., Lambert, E. V., Inoue, S., Ramadan Alkandari, J., Leetongin, G., & Kahlmeier, S. (2012). The pandemic of physical inactivity: Global action for public health. *Lancet*, 380, 294–305. doi:10.1016/S0140-6736(12) 60898-8

Lamb Drover, V. (2014). ParticipACTION, healthism, and the crafting of a social memory (1971–1999). *Journal of the Canadian Historical Association*, 25(1), 277–306. doi:10.7202/1032805ar

Lau, D. C. W., Douketis, J. D., Morrison, K. M., Hramiak, I. M., Sharma, A. M., & Ur, E. (2007). Canadian clinical practice guidelines on the management and prevention of obesity in adults and children [summary]. *Canadian Medical Association Journal*, 176(8), S1–S13.

Le Soleil. (2011). *Kids' gym in Quebec*. Retrieved from www.lepetitgym.ca/

The Little Gym International Inc. (2018). *The little gym*. Retrieved September 2017 from www.thelittlegym.com/our-story#history-anchor

MacDougall, C., Schiller, W., & Darbyshire, P. (2004). We have to live in the future. *Early Child Development and Care*, 174(4), 369–387.

MacNeill, M., & Rail, G. (2010). The visions, voices and moves of young 'Canadians': Exploring diversity, subjectivity and cultural constructions of fitness and health. In J. W. D. Macdonald (Ed.), *Young people, physical activity and the everyday*. New York, NY: Routledge.

Marshall, S. J., Biddle, S. J. H., Gorely, T., Cameron, N., & Murdey, I. (2004). Relationships between media use, body fatness and physical activity in children and youth: A meta-analysis. *International Journal of Obesity*, 28, 1238–1246.

McDermott, L. (2007). A governmental analysis of children 'at risk' in a world of physical inactivity and obesity epidemics. *Sociology of Sport Journal*, 24, 302–324.

McGall, S. E., McGuigan, M. R., & Nottle, C. (2011). Contribution of free play towards physical activity guidelines for New Zealand primary school children aged 7–9 years. *British Journal of Sports Medicine*, 45, 120–124.

McLaren, L., Zarrabi, M., Dutton, D. J., Auld, M. C., & Emery, J. C. (2012). Child care: Implications for overweight/obesity in Canadian children? *Chronic Diseases and Injuries in Canada*, 33(1), 1–11.

Meyer, I. H., & Schwartz, S. (2000). Social issues as public health: Promise and peril. *American Journal of Public Health*, 90(8), 1189–1191.

Mulvihill, C., Rivers, K., & Aggleton, P. (2000). A qualitative study investigating the views of primary-age children and parents on physical activity. *Health Education Journal*, 59, 166–179.

Nadesan, M. (2010). *Governing childhood into the 21st century: Biopolitical technologies of childhood management and education*. New York, NY: Palgrave Macmillan.

O'Loughlin, E. K., Dugas, E. N., Sabiston, C. M., & O'Loughlin, J. L. (2012). Prevalence and correlates of exergaming in youth. *Pediatrics*, 130(5), 806–814.

Onywera, V. O., Héroux, M., Jáuregui Ulloa, E., Adamo, K. B., Taylor, J. L., Janssen, I., & Tremblay, M. S. (2013). Adiposity and physical activity among children in countries at different stages of the physical activity transition: Canada, Mexico and Kenya. *African Journal for Physical, Health Education, Recreation and Dance, 19*(1), 132–142.

Parliament of Canada. (2007). *Healthy weights for healthy kids: Report of the standing committee on health.* Ottawa, Canada: House of Commons Committee, 39th Parliament, 1st Session. Retrieved from www.parl.gc.ca/HousePublications/Publication.aspx?DocId=2795145&File=9

ParticipACTION. (2011a). *Get moving – Active ways to play!* Toronto: ParticipACTION.

ParticipACTION. (2011b). *ParticipACTION toolkit: Think again.* Retrieved June 2011 from http://toolkit.participaction.com/details/en/?asset_id=116

ParticipACTION. (2012). *Bring back play!* Retrieved July 2012 from www.participaction.com/get-moving/bring-back-play/

ParticipACTION. (2013). *ParticipACTION: Let's get moving.* Retrieved June 2013 from www.participaction.com

ParticipACTION. (2015a). *Impact report 2015: Plays of the year – Our latest achievements as champions of physical activity and sport participation in Canada.* Toronto: ParticipACTION.

ParticipACTION. (2015b). *Healthy, prosperous, united: An active Canada is a better Canada: National policy considerations.* Toronto: ParticipACTION.

PHAC. (2003). *Learning from SARS – Renewal of public health in Canada: A report of the national advisory committee on SARS and public health Ottawa.* Public Health Agency of Canada/Health Canada.

PHAC. (2010). *Physical activity guidelines.* Retrieved October 2010 from www.phac-aspc.gc.ca/hp-ps/hl-mvs/pa-ap/03paap-eng.php

Piggin, J., & Bairner, A. (2016). The global physical inactivity pandemic: An analysis of knowledge production. *Sport, Education and Society, 21*(2), 131–147. doi:10.1080/13573322.2014.882301

Rich, E., Monaghan, L. F., & Aphramor, L. (2010). *Debating obesity: Critical perspectives.* Basingstoke: Palgrave Macmillan.

Rose, N. (1999). *Governing the soul: The shaping of the private self* (2nd ed.). London: Free Association Books.

Russell, W. (2013). Towards a spatial theory of playwork: What can Lefebvre offer as a response to playwork's inherent contradictions? In E. Ryall, W. Russell & M. MacLean (Eds.), *The philosophy of play.* New York, NY: Routledge.

Salmon, J., Ball, K., Crawford, D., Booth, M., Telford, A., Hume, C., . . . Worsley, A. (2005). Reducing sedentary behaviour and increasing physical activity among 10-year-old children: Overview and process evaluation of the 'Switch-Play' intervention. *Health Promotion International, 20*(1), 7–17. doi:10.1093/heapro/dah1502

Skrabanek, P. (1994). *The death of humane medicine and the rise of coercive healthism.* The Social Affairs Unit. Bury St Edmunds, Suffolk: St Edmundsbury Press.

Sharratt, M. T., & Hearst, W. E. (2007). Canada's physical activity guides: Background, process, and development. *Applied Physiology, Nutrition and Metabolism, 32,* S9–S15.

Shayne, R. K., Fogel, V. A., Miltenberger, R. G., & Koehler, S. (2012). The effects of exergaming on physical activity in a third-grade physical education class. *Journal of Applied Behavior Analysis, 45*(1), 211–215.

Shields, M. (2006). Overweight and obesity among children and youth. *Health Reports – Statistics Canada, Canadian Centre for Health Information, 17,* 27–42.

Sport New Zealand. (2013). *Push play campaign.* Retrieved August 2013 from www.sportnz.org.nz/en-nz/communities-and-clubs/Push-Play/

Stephen, R. S. (2006). The consequences of childhood overweight and obesity. *Future Child, 16*(1), 47–67. doi:10.2307/3556550

Sutton-Smith, B. (1995). Conclusion: The persuasive rhetorics of play. In A. D. Pellegrini (Ed.), *The future of play theory: A multidisciplinary inquiry into the contributions of Brian Sutton-Smith* (pp. 275–296). Albany, NY: State University of New York.

Sutton-Smith, B. (1997). *The ambiguity of play.* Boston, MA: Harvard University Press.

Thomson, M., Spence, J. C., Raine, K., & Laing, L. (2008). The association of television viewing with snacking behavior and body weight of young adults. *American Journal of Health Promotion, 22*(5), 329–335. doi:10.4278/ajhp.22.5.329

Tremblay, M. S., Barnes, J. D., & Cowie Bonne, J. (2014). Impact of the active healthy kids Canada report card: A 10-year analysis. *Journal of Physical Activity and Health, 11*(1), S3–S20.

Tremblay, M. S., Gonzalez, S. A., Katzmarzyk, P. T., Onywera, V. O., Reilly, J. J., & Tomkinson, G. (2015). Physical activity report cards: Active healthy kids global alliance and the lancet physical activity observatory. *Journal of Physical Activity and Health, 12*(3), 297–298.

Tremblay, M. S., Gray, C. E., Akinroye, K., Harrington, D. M., Katzmarzyk, P. T., Lambert, E. V., . . . Tomkinson, G. (2014). Physical activity of children: A global matrix of grades comparing 15 countries. *Journal of Physical Activity and Health, 11*(Suppl. 1), S113–S125.

Tremblay, M. S., Kho, M. E., Tricco, A. C., & Duggan, M. (2010). Process description and evaluation of Canadian physical activity guidelines development. *International Journal of Behavioral Nutrition and Physical Activity, 7*(42), 1–16.

Vander Schee, C. J., & Boyles, D. (2010). 'Exergaming,' corporate interests and the crisis discourse of childhood obesity. *Sport, Education and Society, 15*(2), 169–185. doi:10.1080/13573321003683828

Whitlock, E. P., Williams, S. B., Gold, R., Smith, P. R., & Shipman, S. A. (2005). Screening and interventions for childhood overweight: A summary of evidence for the US preventive services task force. *Pediatrics, 116*(1), e125–e144. doi:10.1542/peds.2005-0242

WHO. (2000). *Obesity: Preventing and managing the global epidemic.* Report of a WHO consultation: World Health Organization Technical Report Series (Vol. 894). Geneva, Switzerland: World Health Organization.

WHO. (2004). *Obesity: Preventing and managing the global epidemic.* Geneva, Switzerland: World Health Organization.

WHO. (2010a). *Population-based prevention strategies for childhood obesity: Report of the WHO forum and technical meeting.* Geneva: World Health Organization.

WHO. (2010b). *Global recommendations on physical activity for health.* Geneva, Switzerland: World Health Organisation Press.

WHO. (2012a). *Global strategy on diet, physical activity and health* (Vol. 2012). Geneva, Switzerland: World Health Organization.

WHO. (2012b). *Population-based approaches to childhood obesity prevention.* Geneva, Switzerland: World Health Organisation.

Wright, J., & Harwood, V. (2009). *Biopolitics and the 'Obesity Epidemic': Governing bodies.* New York, NY: Routledge.

Wyatt, S. B., Winters, K. P., & Dubberte, P. M. (2006). Overweight and obesity: Prevalence, consequences, and causes of a growing public health problem. *American Journal of the Medical Sciences, 331*(4), 166–174.

Chapter 4

Playing is fun! (... or is it?)

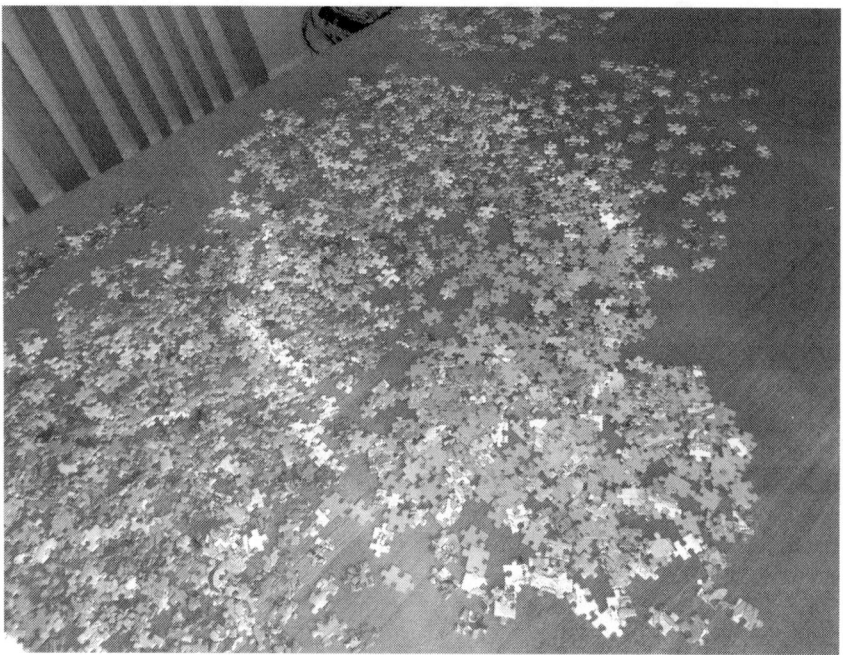

Figure 4.1 Henri (9 years old) took a photo of a puzzle he was working on.

Introduction

Pleasure is a central component of play for children. However, as we have suggested in Chapter 3, depending on how it is framed and promoted, play for children navigates a fine line between pleasure and obligation. In his 1961 book entitled *Man, Play and Games (1961)*, Roger Caillois writes:

> A game which one would be forced to play would at once cease being play. It would become constraint, drudgery from which one would strive to be freed. As an obligation or simply an order, it would lose one of its characteristics. The fact that the player devotes himself spontaneously to the game, of his free will and for his pleasure, each time completely free to choose retreat, silence, meditation, idle solitude or creative activity. It happens only when the players have a desire to play, and play the most absorbing, exhausting game in order to find diversion, escape from responsibility and routine.
> (Caillois, 1961, p. 6)

The pleasure that is often considered to be inherent in play is indeed relatively fragile and can be disrupted by obligation or requirement.

More recently, Twietmeyer (2012) has stated that "[a]lthough, play, games and sports are not magical founts of automatic pleasure production, they do contain the seeds of pleasure" (p. 183). Hackett (2013), more convinced about the pleasurable nature of children's play, argues that play transcends "utilitarian considerations" and that it "brings about the existential satisfaction of restoring ourselves" (p. 124).

Empirical work undertaken with children on the topic of play has found that they generally do not depict their play as fulfilling a particular purpose, goal or outcome. The overriding consensus is that playing involves "fun" (Alexander, Frohlich, & Fusco, 2014; Glenn, Knight, Holt, & Spence, 2012; MacDougall, Schiller, & Darbyshire, 2004), and that conversely, as soon as the activity ceases to be fun (due to any number of reasons), it is no longer considered to be play (Glenn et al., 2012). Summing up the essence of play for children, Sutton-Smith (1997) has argued that play for children, quite simply, "makes them happier" (p. 32).

In our interviews with children we heard similar refrains. One of our participants, Carla, a 10-year-old girl, told us the following about one of the places she liked playing best:

> Well I really like playing there. For me playing is really a break from everything that is, like, disagreeable. Me, I don't like when things are difficult. Often you are like . . . oh! That's hard, I have to work, but I will get there. But playing, it's really a break, you have fun, so I really like it. I feel good when I play.

As we have discussed in previous chapters, however, it appears that the pleasure and fun in children's play is at risk of being transformed through the public health concern with children's physical activity. While the notions of pleasure and fun in fact figure largely in the public health literature regarding children's physical activity promotion, they are prescribed in specific ways. The public health discourse endorses a highly governed form of play that is assumed to be pleasurable for children: play that is physically active, healthy and is deemed safe.

But play has not always been under the gaze of public health. As we learned in Chapter 3, public health institutions have addressed play, a children's social practice that was formerly extrinsic to public health concerns, and brought it within the realm of public health because of the assumed link between changes in children's play and the rise in obesity. Some argue that this link has been used as a moral battleground over children's bodies (Rail, 2012; Wellard, 2012; Wright & Harwood, 2009). Aligning with the ideologies of neo-liberalism, in which individuals are made responsible for their own health (Lupton, 1995), within this new form of morality play is transformed to mobilise children's physical activity and thus influence their physical health. The valuing of play is in this way reduced to its health consequences and marginalises its implicit value as ungoverned "fun".

How public health prescribes play (and, as we will find, even pleasure in play) is the subject of this chapter. We will discuss the multiple forms of pleasure that health-related activities possess and the ways in which societies over time, and public health in particular, have intervened in these pleasurable activities. We discuss three ways in which pleasure is experienced and understood with respect to health-related practices: 1) pleasure as having fun, enjoying oneself; 2) pleasure in controlling oneself and one's health-related practices and 3) pleasure in being healthy. In this latter form, there is a conflating of pleasure and optimisation of the body. Within this perspective, the pleasure of play is not just about "fun", rather one is meant to find pleasure in being healthy and in becoming a good citizen. This new form of morality is not concerned with denying pleasure, but with encouraging individuals to gain pleasure by doing things for the sake of their physical health. Along these lines, children's play is discussed as pleasurable, but only if it is health-promoting, while the notion of pleasure itself is drawn on in public health discourses to encourage children to play in particular ways. As such, play and its pleasure are "public healthified" (Meyer & Schwartz, 2000), promoted solely for how they can contribute to physical health.

Through this discussion, we trace the history of pleasure and public health and explore the various ways in which pleasure and health have intersected, clashed or overlapped. We begin by drawing on the history of pleasure and public health through the examples of eating, sex, drug-taking and physical activity, exploring the varied ways in which public health has both drawn on and regulated pleasure as a way to govern and control the population's health-related behaviours. We then explore how the public health discourse on pleasure and children's play resembles and differs from discourses of the past, and examine in what ways pleasure in children's play is being reshaped and reimagined through public health actions. We question whether children's play is following a similar fate to multiple other social practices, such as eating, alcohol consumption, sexual practices and smoking cigarettes, all of which are, at their core, pleasurable, but that have been taken up and strictly governed within public health.

Pleasure here can be understood as "jouissance" or as "playful, sensual" (Tinning, 2012). Jouissance involves the pleasures of the body and is experienced through heightened sensualities that have physical, psychic and social connotations that often resist, stand in opposition to or escape the control of culture (Maguire, 2011). Caillois' (1961) concept of "ilinix" describes "moments of pleasure which cause a temporary destruction or disruption of the stability of perception" (Booth, 2009 cited in Wellard, 2012, p. 23). Public health and other health institutions have, over time and due to their mandate of preventing disease and keeping the population healthy, put an inordinate amount of focus on curbing disruptive pleasures and the pleasures involved in these oppositional practices. Pleasure-seeking in relation to many of these practices is viewed to be irrational, irresponsible and, at worst, dangerous.

Hedonic pleasure and the ethics of pleasure

Contemporary discussions of pleasure and its relationship to health and well-being have their roots in Greek philosophy. According to the Greeks there were two distinct routes to the good life – hedonic and eudaimonic. Hedonic understandings are based on the view that the pursuit of pleasure leads to well-being. The eudaimonic view sees pleasure-seeking as limited, with well-being resulting from the quest to potentially forgo hedonistic pleasure in order to construct a life of value. While the former describes idyllic notions of health promotion, the latter can be seen as the forebearer of modern public health approaches in which people are asked to modify their health-relevant consumption and practices in order to attain better health (Thompson & Coveney, 2018).

In 2003, Coveney and Bunton wrote a path-breaking article entitled "In pursuit of the study of pleasure: Implications for health research and practice". It was an original piece for public health researchers given the near absolute silence on the subject of pleasure in public health and within the academy until then. In the text, the authors argued that the origins of many modern public health initiatives have their roots in evangelical, often highly disciplined and religious movements of the 18th and 19th centuries designed to reform unwholesome habits and disruptive behaviours. Within these movements, pleasure was regarded as emotional, or irrational, and Coveney and Bunton (2003) argue that public health sought to replace one form of pleasure (i.e., hedonistic, carnal, libidinal) with another (i.e., aesthetic, ascetic civilised). In effect, they suggest public health can be viewed as a set of attempts to transform pleasurable health-related activities into moral, rational ones.

Coveney (2006) later expands on these ideas in his 2006 book entitled *Food, Morals and Meaning* in which he traces the history of public incursion into nutritional habits and morals. His historical portrait, while focused mainly on nutrition and eating, has many parallels across essential health-related practices, such as physical activity and sex. Furthermore, he explores the trajectory across time of relationships between pleasure and eating through culture and cultural institutions. This foray into the past helps to contextualise public health's incursion into pleasure and how public health discourses around pleasure may "play into" how we understand the role of play in children's lives. By extending this to other health-related social practices, Coveney's interpretation helps us understand how we have come to view our bodies and bodily practices according to a particular kind of morality.

Beginning with Ancient Greece and Rome, Coveney (2006) proposes that where codes of conduct of citizens were dependent on a concern for the appropriate daily management of natural pleasures, including food, eating and sex, moderation of one's pleasure was a key principle. A concern for the self in antiquity was expressed through moderation and self-mastery over one's daily practices. Moderation and self-mastery were not ends in themselves however, as they were considered to enhance pleasure. A specific concern for the self was cultivated through which citizens demonstrated that they could govern their actions. This aesthetics of being, based on a certain form of self-control, led to "truth".

In both Greek and Roman times, Coveney (2006) argues, a balance was sought between what were considered natural pleasures (i.e., eating, drinking alcohol, sexual activity) and the body's needs, uses and desires. Pleasure was the result of the ethical comportment associated with satisfying natural desire in a moderate way. For both the Greeks and the Romans the main concern was the moderation of pleasure – the right amount at the right time – in order to be an ethical citizen. These practices were not viewed as strict moral rules, however; they involved a set of considerations that individuals were to reflect upon. Ethical comportment was therefore a means to pleasure, rather than an ethics delimiting the contours of pleasure.

This type of ethical code of conduct stands in juxtaposition with today's notions of moderation where austerity has replaced moderation as the modus operandi for sculpting pleasure in conduct. For early Christians the problems of food and sex were linked to sins associated with lust and pleasures of the flesh. In distinction from the earlier Greeks and Romans, a range of ethical practices was required for Christians to be rendered pure. Under Christianity, the Church enforced rituals of abstinence such as fasts with the goal of curbing indulgence and thus promoting spirituality. Food and eating were thus designated as practices for which individuals required the exercise of control and self-restraint. The taming of natural desires leading to pleasure was deemed necessary to pursue more important spiritual pursuits, while the human body and its needs were linked to human sensuality and animality. The desired effect of a moral conduct and spiritual purity resulted only from denial and austerity in one's conduct. The outcome was that, for Christians, pleasure was often obtained through extinguishing other forms of pleasure altogether (Coveney, 2006).

According to Pronger (1998), Foucault (1978, 1988, 1990) showed how pleasure is used, and indeed resourced, by socio-cultural discourses and practices. However, Pronger (1998) writes:

> while this resourcing of pleasure has eclipsed the light of Eros, obscured the primordiality of the body, it has not annihilated the sacred possibilities of the body.
>
> (pp. 291–292)

Yet, in modernity, especially in modern sport and games, and as we outline later, even in play, boundaries have been established to control the experiences of the moving body – not unlike those of the enforced rituals of early Christianity. Specifically regarding sport, pleasure has often been linked to homoeroticism and sexuality (Gard & Meyenn, 2000; Pronger, 1999) and thus has been marginalised as a topic of conversation in sport. If pleasure is talked about or made visible in sport, it is most often associated with men taking pleasure in the pain and violence that is enacted in sport spaces (Gard & Meyenn, 2000; Gerdin & Pringle, 2017; Markula & Pringle, 2006). Taking pleasure in winning is also tolerated (Maguire, 2011), as is experiencing pleasure in spectating and in the consumptive practices of sports (Cole & King, 1998; MacNeill, 1998; Miller, 2017). Finding pleasure in being fit and healthy (Gerdin &

Pringle, 2017), and in conforming/being disciplined (Markula & Pringle, 2006; Shogan, 1999) is also valorised. As such Pronger (1998) argues that, in modernity, pleasure and eros are acceptable if they are "properly contained by the appropriate athletic setting, conducted at the appropriate time, within the rules of the game and interpreted as just another contributor to the productive, economic body" (p. 285). Modern sport, and as we argue public health as well, is best served economically and politically when pleasure – and here, pleasure linked to play – is contained and regulated in specific ways.

Controlling pleasure: the danger and risk within

So it is that in 2017 the very foundations of public health thinking and programming are arguably concerned with the disciplining of pleasure. This subtext is inherent in attempts to improve public health: from smoking cessation, improvements in diet, moderation in drinking alcohol and safe sexual practices. The onset of concerns regarding addiction, for example, which began with drug consumption and became a commonplace descriptor for the consequences of tobacco smoking and eating "junk" food, have led to the pathologising of pleasurable behaviours. The discourses around "craving" retain the post-Christian idea of the excesses of the lower orders, and denote that the ability to curb behaviour is beyond an individual's power. Individual behaviour seen in this way is no longer viewed as free-willed pursuit of pleasure, but rather as a failing of the individual to control his/her non-rational side.

We surmise that the heart of the problem for public health is that pleasures challenge self-control. Pleasure in eating, having sex, smoking and, we will argue, playing has become a source of great anxiety. Rather than being interested in the pleasures involved in such activities, public health dictates that the population should be focused on the possibilities for good health that derive from behaving in prescribed ways. The pleasure discourse lacuna in public health is partially due to the fear that discussing it might encourage the continued "excess" (in the Christian sense) of some of the behaviours for which moderation, avoidance, abstinence or eradication is the preferred option (Tinning, 2012; Thompson & Coveney, 2017).

In parallel to being pathologised, pleasure is also often coded as being risky within contemporary public health discourses. Pleasure and pleasure-seeking activities are viewed as being at the root of irrational, often spontaneous actions which predispose individuals to unhealthy, so-called risk-taking behaviours. Within discussions of sports, pleasure-seeking has also frequently been coded as relating to the hedonistic social interactions and party lifestyles of, for instance, snowboarders (Thorpe, 2012), surfers (Booth, 1995) or other extreme/alternative sports (Reinhart, 2014). Reinhart argues that "the pleasure effects of thrill sports – the name itself gives away the sense of it – is the rush, the unwieldy loss of control, perhaps the seeming pushing of limits" (p. 11). These kinds of sports have historically "generated anxiety among a moralistic middle class intent on disciplining youth" (Booth, 1995, p. 206). While people, particularly youth, continue to engage in extreme sports, they are often marginalised in spaces where they can be contained (Borden, 2001), or discussions of these sports are couched in language about risk and injury, which, not surprisingly, emanates from public health- and morality-based discursive incursions into physical culture (Rail, 2012).

Returning to public health discourses, sexual practices and pleasure-seeking activities among gay men, for example, have been linked to unprotected, ergo unsafe, sex (Coveney & Bunton, 2003). This equation of pleasure with risk is particularly problematic, specifically in the areas of drug harm reduction and the prevention of sexually transmitted diseases. Ignoring the inherent human pleasures of drug-taking and having sex, however, has also proven to be problematic, particularly given the relatively recent acknowledgement that pleasure must be accommodated for in harm reduction programmes and policies, otherwise they risk failure. Examples occur in the ways that abstinence narratives have given way to harm minimisation in the fields of sex education, the management of HIV among men who have sex with men, in relation to the use of "hard" drugs and needle exchanges and, increasingly, with regard to tobacco smoking. Harm reduction policy and practice attempts to construct a particular form of individual – a health-conscious person capable of rational decision-making, self-regulation and risk management. However, adopting this concept of the neo-liberal subject ignores attributes that do not sit comfortably with alternative views of people as pleasure and desire seekers. Indeed, even these harm-minimising discourses ignore the strong and fundamental relationship between health-related activities and pleasure (O'Malley & Valverde, 2004); they simply constitute a pragmatic response in the face of resistance to, or lack of efficacy of, prior public health interventions.

With respect to physical education, Wellard (2012) argues that "[t]he lack of exploration about 'what fun is', may in part be explained by the association of fun with subjective pleasure and the consequent risks of being drawn into debates about hedonism" (p. 30), which is linked to individual notions of pleasure. Interesting recent work on sexual education suggests that pleasure was used in a way to bolster talk about safety only, but not to discuss pleasure in its own right. Surprisingly, pleasure in discussions of sexual health (Lamb, Lustig, & Galing, 2013) was introduced in order to address the topics of risk, self-control, regrettable sex and peer pressure. Pleasure therefore tends to be discussed negatively with a focus on danger and risk-prevention or as an obstacle to restraint, abstinence and health rather than as something meant to enhance self-knowledge, as a fun activity, as a way to get to know someone etc.

Elias and Dunning (1986) argued quite some time ago that "a principal function of leisure is the 'arousal of pleasurable forms of excitement'" (in Maguire, 2011, p. 919). However, as within public health, in the fields of physical activity and physical education, there has been an absence of discussions of this kind of pleasure, with the notable exception of Featherstone (1991) and McKay, Gore, and Kirk (1990). Pleasure or desire was not central to any discussions of physical education, except negatively, where physical education was constructed as strategic in the control of desire (the desire to indulge in delicious, but harmful and fattening foods) (Pronger, 2002, pp. 7–8). While the notion of pleasure was viewed as problematic (especially in early Christian and Victorian times), it was sport and recreation, particularly for young men, that resulted in the ethos of "pleasure-rightly used" (Erdozain, 2010) – that is, a good dose of gymnastics, sports and recreation would be the means by which character-building could occur and dangerous temptations avoided. More recently, however, Gerdin and Pringle's (2017) work expands the growing body of literature in studies of physical education and pleasure (see Gard & Meyenn, 2000; Tinning, 2012; Twietmeyer, 2012; Wellard, 2012). In their ethnographic study of the physical education classes at an all-boys secondary school in Aotearoa, New Zealand, Gerdin and Pringle (2017) explore the idea that the sensual pleasures the boys voiced with regard to their fitness classes is evidence of the discursive conjunction between health, fitness and physical activity. This conjunction creates a feeling of moral goodness amongst the boys that they are "doing the right thing" by being physically active. The authors argue that the boys' feelings about their involvements in sport was shaped by the health discourses of their teachers and that the boys were being taught to understand the pleasures inherent in believing that they were taking individual responsibility for their own health and well-being through participation in the physical education classes.

While embodied feelings of movement and mobility can engender intense pleasures and sensuous feelings, in an era of public health governance of leisure activities, and exercise as medicine and corporeal therapeutics (Fullagar, 2017), "pleasure remains largely unspoken and dangerous territory" (Gard & Meyenn, 2000, p. 19). Pleasure is important, but it remains a neglected and often misunderstood aspect of kinesiology, sport and physical activity (Twietmeyer, 2012).

Can play still be frivolous pleasure?

What does this all have to do with children's play? Play as a social and recently circumscribed health-related practice does not naturally fall within the usual suspect list of potentially nefarious health behaviours such as drug-taking, unprotected sex, eating (indulging in) unhealthy foods, heavy alcohol consumption and tobacco smoking. But play is not immune to the overall public health discourse on pleasure, which views purely pleasurable activities as somehow risky.

We explore the onset of discussions within public health of children's play as both a science and a morality, and view children's play as potentially mapping onto the concerns that public health has regarding other health-related behaviours. Furthermore, while children's play is, in principle, not a practice that can be seen as risky or dangerous (differently from drug consumption, tobacco smoking, poor dietary habits, excess consumption of alcohol and unprotected sex), there is a definitive tendency over the last 10 years of discussing play in surprisingly similar terms.

For instance, while Canadian parents have recently been asked to loosen their once protective grip on their children's play, allowing children to take more risks and simply enjoy their play, parents are also charged with producing new risks for children. The 2012 Report Card suggests:

> The net result of our over-parenting behaviours is decreased physical activity, decreased fresh air and sunlight exposure, increased obesity and increased risk of harm from cyber-crime.
>
> (AHKC, 2012, p. 24)

There are aspects to this discourse that are novel in relation to the other health-related behaviours previously discussed. First, the discourse is about pleasure and children, rather than adults. Disciplining of the child and his/her social life is somewhat new, although, as we will see in greater detail in Chapter 5, it is both the children and their families that require self-disciplining in order to play appropriately. Second, pleasure in children's play can actually serve a purpose. Differently from the pleasure conferred from sex, cigarette smoking and drug-taking, which is seen as either uniquely irrational or generally frivolous, pleasure in play is both seen as frivolous (purposeless), but also as an opportunity to do something morally good – to be healthy and assist in optimal development (as we discussed in Chapter 2).

As Tinning (2012) has argued, the quest for a healthy citizen is a tug-of-war in which different vested interests compete for the hearts and minds of young people. But the concerns about risk and danger remain, dragging the discourse on pleasure in play down a path towards its marginalisation and denial. Indeed, the Canadian grey literature on play and physical activity has demonstrated both a strong tendency to instrumentalise play, suggesting that it is a potentially frivolous and dangerous activity if simply engaged in for pleasure. For instance, CSEP's physical activity *Guidelines* have been drawn on by ParticipACTION and AHKC to suggest that children who are not active enough are potentially precipitating an obesity epidemic. It is precisely in the construction of 'inactive children' as a central problem that the relevance of children's play activities enters the field of public health. As the 2011 AHKC (2011) Report Card notes, children's "modern" leisure activities are particularly problematic:

> Anecdotally, we know that most children who grew up a generation or two ago spent this time in active play, running, biking and playing (usually outside) with their friends. Various data sources suggest that this is not the case today; Canadian children and youth have adopted a modern lifestyle that includes spending a great deal of this after-school time sitting idle indoors.
>
> (p. 3)

Even though it has been debated whether modern children are in fact less active than those of previous generations, what is relevant is that the explicit problem (that is, children's obesity epidemic) carries within it an implicit problem: that of the leisure pursuits of inactive children. This implicit problem is further highlighted and reinforced by the solutions formulated to address it: workbooks and media releases address the *Guidelines* by promoting "active play" to children (as discussed in Chapter 3) (Alexander, Frohlich, & Fusco, 2015). As AHKC (2010, p. 3) suggests: "at least half of the physical activity accumulated by children should be through active play".

The promotion of children's active play thus underscores the implicit problem of "idle" children with modern-day, inactive lifestyles, and the increasing threat of obesity reinforces the desire to subject children's leisure activities to urgent modification. As discussed in Chapter 3, a discourse on active play has begun to take form, framed as an ideal leisure activity and solution to the problem of the children's obesity crisis. Unfortunately, such a perspective means that the potential for bodily pleasures experienced through physical activity and play become managed within particular social and health discourses (Wellard, 2012). Indeed, the requirement that play be productive remains relatively unchallenged in this discourse. Within these parameters it appears unacceptable – even irresponsible – to promote play without an explicit productive purpose (for example, to promote play for pleasure alone). Playing requires justification to lend legitimacy to its promotion in public health. As suggested by ParticipACTION (2012):

> Active play may be lots of fun for youngsters, but it's certainly not frivolous . . . it is also shown to improve a child's motor function, creativity, decision-making, problem-solving and social skills.

Furthermore, the social and economic consequences attributed to children's obesity reinforce the importance of active play, directly linking children's play and their pleasure to the social and economic prosperity of the country. Thus, within the public health discourse, play is a rather serious activity for children, and it appears that other dimensions of play, such as the social and the relational dimensions, and those elements that are simply fun, have been neglected (Downward & Dawson, 2016).

Several assumptions about the relationship between pleasure and physical activity emerge in this discourse. One notable element concerns the way in which pleasure functions as a trope for physical activity. Indeed, as suggested earlier, pleasure and fun are drawn upon within public health to promote active play and are assumed to be essential components of physical activity for all children. For instance, ParticipACTION's 2011 workbook *Active Ways to Play!* implies that being active and having fun necessarily coexist for children (Alexander et al., 2015). They propose to children: "Hey kids, this is your free time, and your only job is to make it active and to have fun" (p. 3). Such assertions about pleasure, physical activity and obesity culminate in conclusions such as: "the direction to go and play more after school should be a welcome prescription for a healthy active life for our children" (AHKC, 2011, p. 2). Under such circumstances, the rational health approach is privileged over the embodied, sensual and non-rational dimensions of children's play experiences, with little consideration for the pleasure that is intrinsic to play (Tinning, 2012).

These statements not only assume that fun and pleasure are the qualities experienced by all children who engage in physical activity, but that by prescribing play as a proxy for physical activity they also underscore the function of play (and its pleasure) as a health practice (Alexander et al., 2014). Wellard (2012) argues that "[t]hrough time a restricted rhetoric of health, if constantly extolled . . . will further alienate many individuals from their bodies" (p. 31). He continues:

> for many young people and adults with limited experience or enthusiasm for sport, the physical aspects of bodily pleasure are often overlooked in favour of specific health-related measures. The implication being that the motivation for taking part is, for example, to lose weight with the consequence that their introduction (and subsequent orientation) to sport and physical activity is related to a specific outcome – rather than as an enjoyable embodied experience.
>
> (p. 23)

Given that fun and pleasure are conceived of as important elements of children's physical activity, parents and guardians are given the responsibility of providing children with frequent opportunities for physical activity that children will enjoy. For instance, ParticipACTION (2010, p. 1) encourages parents and guardians to "make physical activity a fun, regular part of everyday", while the Public Health Agency of Canada (PHAC) (2008) educates parents on the importance of reinforcing pleasure as a primary motivator for physical activity (Alexander et al., 2014). They write:

> Although physical activity results in many health benefits, these benefits do not motivate young people to be physically active. Rather, they tend to participate in physical activity for fun and enjoyment, and for social reasons.
>
> (p. 39)

Moreover, as a further responsibility to their children, parents and guardians are expected themselves to adopt a positive disposition towards physical activity; one that takes similar pleasure in being active (Alexander et al., 2014). Indeed, parents and guardians are encouraged to show explicit enjoyment of physical activity for the sake of their children's health. As a cogent example, ParticipACTION (2010) recommends to parents and guardians:

> Be a good role model. Make sure you live an active life. It's important for your kids to see you running, walking, playing sports regularly

after work. Display a positive attitude that being active is fun and feels good.

(p. 46)

The discourse thus appears to place a dual responsibility on parents and guardians. Not only should they "get their kids active" for health purposes, but they are expected to ensure that the activity is fun for the sake of their child's future enjoyment of (and investment in) physical activity (Alexander et al., 2014). As we argued previously (Alexander et al., 2014), "parents and guardians who do not (or cannot) take up these prescriptions, and who do not (or cannot) engage in physical activities (while feigning pleasure and enjoyment) are nonetheless unrelentingly reminded of their duty to be involved in the provision of fun, active play for their child's wellbeing" (p. 1196). AHKC (2010) asks parents and guardians:

> What are YOU doing to provide opportunities for children to engage in free, unstructured, active play? Do YOU encourage, promote and participate in active outdoor play?
>
> (p. 10)

Thus, the concepts of fun and pleasure as they relate to play are closely bound to the promotion of physical activities for children based on the assumption that play is necessarily active, and that active forms of playing will necessarily be fun for all children (Alexander et al., 2014). Parents and guardians are not only made responsible for reinforcing these associations (that fun equates physical activity) but for modelling this enjoyment themselves.

Early intervention through educating children about healthy lifestyles emerges as a significant preventive health measure and is viewed as a means to ensure that children are set on a path to future health and well-being. ParticipACTION's workbooks, for instance, are created to encourage children to learn to evaluate their own active play and assign an academic grade based on how many minutes they have been playing actively. The workbook suggests to parents:

> Have your kids track their daily physical activity. At the end of the week, see how many days they've hit 60 minutes per day. Use the handy chart to assign a weekly mark. Get ready, set, go! Look for the activity tracker on the back page of the after-school activity guide. Post

one for each child in the house and see who can have the most fun getting an *A*.

(ParticipACTION, 2011, p. 2)

What is being promoted is a very specific kind of pleasure for a particular child subject: a child who can govern his/her healthy lifestyle according to public health prescriptions and, most importantly, who takes pleasure in playing actively.

These kinds of discourses are not surprising in an era of neo-liberal political and economic realities. Children and parents are supposed to gain pleasure from adhering to public health mandates, and the neo-liberal rational works in such a way that individuals gain pleasure precisely from participating in and being a healthy citizen (Gerdin & Pringle, 2017). As Lupton (1995) so deftly argues:

> The self that is being privileged and normalized in such discourses is that of the enterprising and entrepreneurial self, the individual who is interested in and willing to take action to improve his or her health status. It is assumed that all individuals have the potential for such social action in the name of good health, and that it is simply up to the health promotion officer to encourage or "facilitate" the realization of this potential.
>
> (p. 61)

To paraphrase Donzelot (1991), who critiqued how neo-liberal/capitalist regimes produced the ideology of pleasure through work in the interests of greater efficiency and lesser cost (p. 280), children's play in current public health agendas appears to be "in response to malaise caused in pursuit of productivity/good citizenship, intended to make [play] as a good in itself, a means towards self-realization" (p. 255). A lack of pleasure in active play then would be seen as a "moral rupture which precipitates the demoralization of society" (Donzelot, p. 258). Similarly, Gerdin and Pringle (2017) have suggested that systems of thought and mechanisms of power shape how humans experience, understand and manage pleasure. It is therefore essential that public health be cognizant of the shaping of the idea of what pleasurable play is and should be.

Pringle, Rinehart, and Caudwell (2015) have recently examined the social significance of pleasure and sport and the notion of government-regulated pleasure, in which subjective well-being and physical activity participation are brought under the control of government. In the same way, the concepts of fun and pleasure in play are closely bound to the promotion of physical activities for children based on the assumption that play is necessarily active, and that active forms of playing will necessarily be fun for all children. Parents and guardians are not only made responsible for reinforcing these associations (that fun equates physical activity), but for modelling this enjoyment themselves.

When the pleasure is gone

The instrumentalisation of children's play, and in some cases its commodification, risks changing children's experiences of their playing. Reflecting back on the ParticipACTION workbooks, Tinning (2012) might argue that "[t]he jouissance which children derived from consumer culture is designed to ensure that they unreflexively consume rather than interpret such texts" (p. 75). Pronger (2002) similarly suggests in his writings about modern sport:

> There is pleasure in sport; there is ecstasy in a good run, a hard swim, cycling up a hill against a wind. The modern reading of that pleasure casts it in socio-cultural discourses of competitive sport. . . . The experience of ecstasy (the de-eclipsing of the sacred) doesn't always take a postmodern turn. This is not surprising given that there is little or no encouragement for such a turn in our physical culture. Certainly, sport does not encourage it. And physical fitness culture is more about the forever unrequited pleasure of consumption, or the instrumentality of the physically active body in the production of economically viable bodies and the shaping of body surfaces along fashionable socio-cultural lines, than it is about the postmodern experience of embodiment.
>
> (pp. 292–293)

Indeed, as the discourse around children's play becomes increasingly commodified and linked explicitly to health outcomes, the notion that play and physical activity can be fun and engaged in to "just feel good" may even be lost (Wright & Macdonald, 2010). As we outlined in Chapter 3, inherent in the somewhat paradoxical message in which children are encouraged to track, tabulate and govern their play while also ensuring that it is fun, is the message that active play is akin to schoolwork. By drawing a parallel between the competition and evaluation of academic work and children's self-government of active play, children's play becomes linked with academic achievement. Under these circumstances, active play as a governed and evaluated activity appears to relate very little (or at best indirectly) to fun and enjoyment and remains quite distant from the unstructured pleasure that children are simultaneously being encouraged to gain from their active forms of play (Alexander et al., 2014). Furthermore, this perspective assumes that all children will find competition in play rewarding and that all children will find pleasure in active play. It is taken for granted that the competitive evaluation of play activities is a notion to which all children will excitedly relate and, importantly, a value that all families share (Alexander et al., 2014).

But these instrumental notions of pleasure in play clash considerably with the actual notions of fun and "unrequited pleasure" (Pronger, 2002) of play that our participants voiced. Take for example Sarah, an 11-year-old girl who participated in our study. When we asked her to describe what she finds fun in play, she responded:

> It's a soccer net and we just shoot goals in it and around it. It's fun because we don't really play it by the rules. We always end up falling on the ground and talking.

So while current advocates of active play might celebrate this girl's active use of her time playing soccer, the real pleasure in her play comes from not really playing by the rules, but rather from engaging in various kinds of play, some of which are active, others of which are not (i.e., "falling on the ground and talking").

By regulating children's play to be healthy and active, and thus normalising the ways in which children are encouraged to play, other relevant qualities of play may be also neglected. Indeed, while playing simply for fun (that is, frivolous pleasure) is considered a common experience of childhood, it appears to be less important than the more productive and explicitly active play for health. Considering the discourse from a child's vantage point, the forms of play mandated by public health – those prescribed to be healthy, active, monitored, tabulated and evaluated – play becomes an activity engendering qualities decidedly different from forms of leisure that are more freely chosen. Eric, a 7-year-old boy participating in our study, described his favourite ways of playing in the following way:

> Building lego. That's what I like the most. You can destroy them and then rebuild them. Because you can always redo them. You destroy it, you can redo it. You destroy it, you can redo it. OK, it never stops. Sometimes I get dizzy 'cause I have done this so much.

This description of a play activity in which the pleasure or fun comes from its repetitious nature – to "destroy it" and "redo it" – may appear to adults as frivolity, pointless, unproductive. Yet the possibility for repeating an activity, playing with it and its continuity are what make this pleasurable play for this boy.

Alain, an 11-year-old boy, discusses a favourite way of playing that involves the management of pleasure and risk in the playground at school:

> Say, you know the little carousel . . . the carousel is about 1 meter, or maybe even 3 meters high at one point, and sometimes we jump off of it and try to do moves in the air. And at one point someone got hurt doing that. They got caught on something jumping down and they hurt their leg. But up until now, it hasn't happened to me. . . . I like doing this, but I wouldn't say you could do it necessarily every day, whenever. Because in the summer I wouldn't do it for sure. And in the fall, even if there are leaves, it's not thick enough. And in the winter, what I like, is that on top of having your thick jacket and snow pants for jumping and all that, and even when we don't have our snow pants, well, there's snow to catch our fall. So, in the end, there's no risk really to get hurt.

This form of pleasure (a form of active play) involves the risk of injury, as his friend experienced, and is generally prohibited by the school staff. By continuing to play this way requires experience with the form of play (i.e., when to do it and when not to do it), as well as a negotiation of the way the potential risks of injury can be managed in order to not evacuate the thrilling pleasure of jumping off of a 3-metre-high play structure.

Taken together, we suggest that the interrogation of this emerging discourse in public health is especially important, as it underscores the need to recognise that the discourse on healthy active play, with its instrumentalisation, may foreclose speaking about pleasure in a way that opens a window onto the power of the visceral, corporeal and non-rational pleasures (Tinning, 2012). Similarly, there is evidence, for instance, that when physical education is focused on physical fitness, instead of physical activity for fun, children are less likely to enjoy it (Gard & Wright, 2005; Wellard, 2012). Although children may find a great deal of pleasure in activities that are defined by adults as healthy, it is altogether possible that children may resent the anxieties being foisted upon them to engage in activities that are explicitly "fat burning", rather than just purely physically pleasurable. Wellard (2012) argues that we need to recognise the range of pleasures available in sport and physical activity in order to be able to promote positive (pleasurable) experiences for young people – so that they can reflect and make decisions about further participation.

This kind of agency – that our 11-year-old participant discusses in his risky play – appears to be lacking in the public health promotion of active play. Pronger (1998) would argue that a postmodern pleasure paradigm is vital to the recovery of pleasure and eros in sports, games and, we would add, play. He states:

> physical activity needs to play with the pleasure of chaos. This will be an innovative, educational form of erotic play whose anarchic, indeed wild tendencies are both socially/psychically dangerous and full of positive potential – because it brings people to the edge of the existential abyss that lies just beyond the confines of modernity.
>
> (p. 293)

In the latest twist of the public health incursion into play, there has been, over the last 3 to 5 years, new messaging to parents and children in Canada about risky and dangerous play, but rather than prohibiting it, it is explicitly encouraged as fun; less regulation and more outdoor and free-ranging play is required. Indeed, the latest statements on active outdoor play suggest that play *should* be *risky* (emphasis added). Might this be a turn to the pleasure paradigm that Pronger (1998) argues for? Or is this new policy on risky play a re-inscription of neo-liberal enterprises "for socially mobilizing individuals towards saving in the cost of healthcare and collaboration in their pursuit?" (Donzelot, 1991, p. 279). It is to this subject of risky play that we turn to in the next chapter.

References

Active Healthy Kids Canada. (2010). *The active healthy kids Canada report card on physical activity for children and youth*. Toronto, Canada: Active Health Kids Canada.

Active Healthy Kids Canada. (2011). *Today's after school special – Inactivity: Canadian children missing the mark on physical activity in the after-school period*. Toronto, Canada: Active Health Kids Canada.

Active Healthy Kids Canada. (2012). *Is active play extinct? Report card on physical activity for children and youth*. Toronto, Canada: Active Health Kids Canada. Retrieved from www.activehealthykids.ca/ReportCard/ArchivedReportCards.aspx

Alexander, S. A., Frohlich, K. L., & Fusco, C. (2014). 'Active play may be lots of fun. . . . but it's certainly not frivolous': The emergence of active play as a health practice in Canadian public health. *Sociology of Health and Illness*, 36(8), 1188–1204.

Alexander, S. A., Frohlich, K. L., & Fusco, C. (2015). 'You have to do 60 minutes of physical activity per day! I saw it on TV': Children's experiences of playing

within the context of the public health discourse of playing for health. *Sociology of Health and Illness, 37*(2), 227–240.
Booth, D. (1995). Ambiguities in pleasures and discipline: The development of competitive surfing. *Journal of Sports History, 22*(3), 189–206.
Booth, D. (2009). Politics and pleasure: The philosophy of physical education revisited. *Quest, 61,* 133–153.
Borden, I. (2001). *Skateboarding, space and the city: Architecture and the body.* Oxford: BERG.
Caillois, R. (1961). *Man, play and games.* Urbana and Chicago, IL: University of Illinois Press.
Cole, C., & King, S. (1998). Representing black masculinity and urban possibilities: Racism, Realism, and hoop dreams. In G. Rail (Ed.), *Sport and postmodern times* (pp. 49–86). Albany, NY: SUNY Press.
Coveney, J. (2006). *Food, morals and meaning: The pleasure and anxiety of eating* (2nd ed.). London: Routledge.
Coveney, J., & Bunton, R. (2003). In pursuit of the study of pleasure: Implications for health research and practice. *Health: An Interdisciplinary Journal for the Social Study of Health, Illness and Medicine, 7*(2), 161–179.
Donzelot, J. (1991). The mobilization of society. In G. Burchell, C. Gordon & P. Miller (Eds.), *The Foucault effect: Studies in governmentality* (pp. 169–180). Chicago, IL: The University of Chicago Press.
Downward, P., & Dawson, P. (2016). Is it pleasure or health from leisure that we benefit from most? An analysis of well-being alternatives and implications for policy. *Social Indicators Research, 126*(1), 443–465.
Elias, N., & Dunning, E. (1986). *Quest for excitement: Sport and leisure in the civilising process.* Oxford: Basil Blackwell.
Erdozain, D. (2010). *The problem of pleasure: Sport, recreation and the crisis of Victorian religion.* Woodbridge, UK: Boydell Press.
Featherstone, M. (1991). *Consumer culture and postmodernism.* London: Sage Publications.
Foucault, M. (1978). *The history of sexuality* (Vol. 1). New York, NY: Random House.
Foucault, M. (1988). *The care of the self: The history of sexuality* (Vol. 3, R. Hurley, Trans.). New York, NY: Vintage Books.
Foucault, M. (1990). *The use of pleasure: The history of sexuality* (Vol. 2, R. Hurley, Trans.). New York, NY: Vintage Books.
Fullagar, S. (2017). Mind-body relations in physical cultural studies: Exploring the rise of a new corporeal therapeutics in mental health. In M. Silk, D. Andrews & H. Thorpe (Eds.), *The Routledge handbook of physical cultural studies.* London: Routledge.
Gard, M., & Meyenn, R. (2000). Boys, bodies, pleasure and pain: Interrogating contact sports in schools. *Sport, Education and Society, 5*(1), 19–34.
Gard, M., & Wright, J. (2005). *The obesity epidemic: Science, morality, and ideology.* New York, NY: Routledge.
Gerdin, G., & Pringle, R. (2017). The politics of pleasure: An ethnographic examination exploring the dominance of the multi-activity sport-based physical education model. *Sport, Education and Society, 22*(2), 194–213.
Glenn, N. M., Knight, C. J., Holt, N. L., & Spence, J. C. (2012). Meanings of play among children. *Childhood, 20*(2), 185–199.

Hackett, T. (2013). Passion play, free will and the sublime. In E. Ryall, W. Russell & M. MacLean (Eds.), *The philosophy of play* (pp. 120–129). London: Routledge.

Lamb, S., Lustig, K., & Galing, K. (2013). The use and misuse of pleasure in sex education curricula. *Sex Education, 13*(3), 305–318.

Lupton, D. (1995). *The imperative of public health: Public health and the regulated body.* London: Sage Publications.

MacDougall, C., Schiller, W., & Darbyshire, P. (2004). We have to live in the future. *Early Child Development and Care, 174*(4), 369–387.

MacNeill, M. (1998). Sex, lies, and videotape: The political and cultural economies of celebrity fitness videos. In G. Rail (Ed.), *Sport and postmodern times* (pp. 163–184). Albany, NY: SUNY Press.

Maguire, J. (2011). Welcome to the pleasure dome: Emotions, leisure and society. *Sport in Society, 4*(7/8), 913–926.

Markula, P., & Pringle, R. (2006). *Foucault, sport and exercise: Power, knowledge and transforming the self.* London: Routledge.

McKay, J., Gore, J., & Kirk, D. (1990). Beyond the limits of technocratic physical education. *Quest, 42*(1), 52–75.

Meyer, I. H., & Schwartz, S. (2000). Social issues as public health: Promise and peril. *American Journal of Public Health, 90*(8), 1189–1191.

Miller, T. (2017). Spectacular and eroticized bodies. In M. Silk, D. Andrews & H. Thorpe (Eds.), *Handbook of physical cultural studies* (pp. 246–256). New York, NY: Routledge.

O'Malley, P., & Valverde, M. (2004). Pleasure, freedom and drugs: The uses of 'pleasure' in liberal governance of drug and alcohol consumption. *Sociology, 38*(1), 25–42.

ParticipACTION. (2010). *Tips on how to get your young children to move more.* Available at content/uploads/2013/09/activehealthykidscanada2010-participaction tipssheet.pdf (accessed 20 April 2011).

ParticipACTION. (2011). *Think again campaign.* Retrieved June 2012 from www.youtube.com/watch?v=GM7HY2HqXEI&list=PLn9ck0OZhxkYVlk_itMNGnDdS5pqmcTOX&index=6

ParticipACTION. (2012). *Bring back play!* Retrieved from www.participaction.com/get-moving/bring-back-play-1/

Pringle, R., Rinehart, R. E., & Caudwell, J. (2015). *Sport and the social significance of pleasure.* London: Routledge.

Pronger, B. (1998). Post-sport: Transgressing boundaries in physical culture. In G. Rail (Ed.), *Sport and postmodern times: Culture, gender, sexuality, the body and sport.* Buffalo, NY: SUNY.

Pronger, B. (1999). Outta my endzone: Sport and the territorial anus. *Journal of Sport & Social Issues, 23*(4), 373–389.

Pronger, B. (2002). *Body fascism: Salvation in the technology of physical fitness.* Toronto: University of Toronto Press.

Public Health Agency of Canada (PHAC). (2008). *Healthy settings for young people in Canada.* Ottawa, Canada: Health Canada.

Rail, G. (2012). The birth of the obesity clinic: Confessions of the flesh, biopedagogies and physical culture. *Sociology of Sport Journal, 29*(2), 227–253.

Reinhart, R. (2014). Anhedonia and alternative sports. *Staps, 2*(104), 9–21. doi:10.3917/sta.104.0009

Shogan, D. (1999). *The making of high performance athletes: Discipline, diversity, and ethics*. Toronto: University of Toronto Press.

Sutton-Smith, B. (1997). *The ambiguity of play*. Boston, MA: Harvard University Press.

Thompson, L., & Coveney, J. (2017). Human vulnerabilities, transgression and pleasure. *Critical Public Health*, 28(1), 118–128. doi:10.1080/09581596.2017.1309356

Thorpe, H. (2012). 'Sex, drugs, and snowboarding': (Il)legitimate definitions of taste and lifestyle in a physical youth culture. *Leisure Studies*, 3(1), 31–51.

Tinning, R. (2012). The idea of physical education: A memetic perspective. *Physical Education and Sport Pedagogy*, 17(2), 115–126.

Twietmeyer, G. (2012), The merits and demerits of pleasure in kinesiology. *Quest*, 64, 177–186.

Wellard, I. (2012). Body-reflexive pleasures: Exploring bodily pleasure within the context of sport and physical activity. *Sport, Education and Society*, 17(1), 21–33.

Wright, J., & Harwood, V. (Eds.). (2009). *Biopolitics and the obesity epidemic: Governing bodies*. Oxon, UK: Routledge.

Wright, J., & Macdonald, D. (2010). *Young people, physical activity and the everyday*. London: Routledge.

Chapter 5

Risk, play and free-range kids

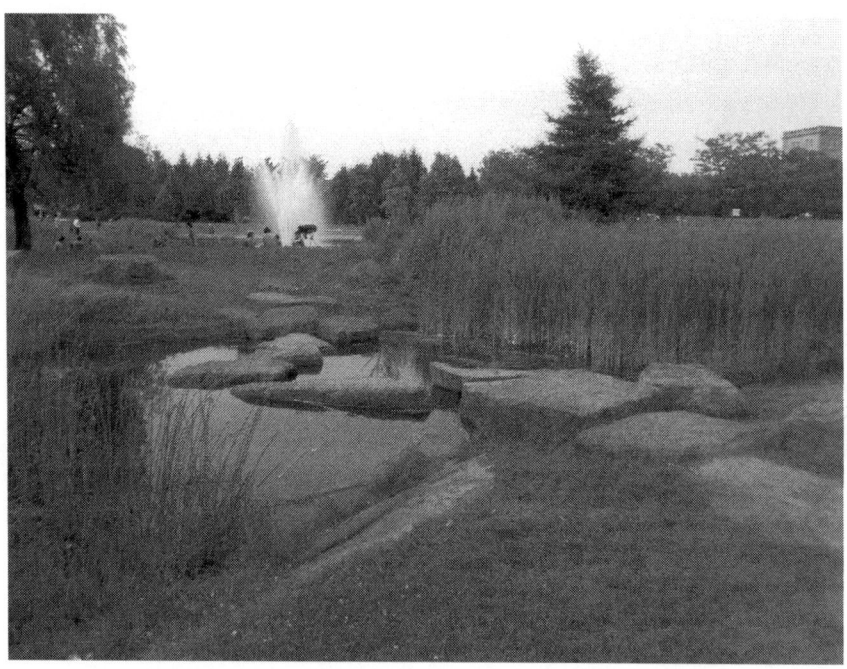

Figure 5.1 Lisette (7 years old) took a photo of her favourite place in a park.

Introduction

Understanding risk and pleasure as two sides of the same coin (Coveney & Bunton, 2003), this chapter moves to a discussion of risk in children's play. We outline the development of a "culture of fear" around childhood generally, and the inundation of risk narratives around children's leisure activities specifically with respect to children's movement and independent mobility, playgrounds and risk, parental and child responsibility for the risks assumed in not playing (e.g., the perils of electronics, bad indoor air) and the new norm of acceptable risk in playing outside.

Indeed, there has been an interesting trajectory of beliefs and concerns. For instance, taking any risks as part of play was to be avoided at all cost. Children's physical safety (i.e., an absence of all physical harm) has been of foremost importance, and for many families with young children it almost seems subversive, irresponsible and legally questionable to conceive of playing as having some form of physical risk. As such, play in some contexts is still increasingly defined through risk and safety (Cooper, 2000; Frost, 2010). Yet, there have been some contradictions creeping into public health discussions around risk and play: on the one hand it is suggested that physical activity can be risky, on the other hand, the discourse also points to the risk of not playing actively enough (as outlined in previous chapters). Some researchers and play advocates argue for the necessity to include risk in children's lives and in their play activities, and there is even a movement to encourage "free-range kids", and for children to take back the streets and nature.

In this chapter, we will discuss some of this literature on risk and play. The different discourses around risk and play often dovetail with discourses of criminalisation (e.g., of those who allow their children too much freedom) and responsibilisation (e.g., of those who do not allow their children enough freedom to play). Into these contradictory and competing discourses, public health has weighed in with its recommendations for risk and play through their promotion of "outdoor active play".

Framing risk

In the last 30 years, risk discourses about many of our social practices have proliferated because some have argued we live in what has been called a "risk society", where the prevention and minimization of (bad) risks have become a central focus (Beck, 1992). Risk, once seen as part of the natural processes of life, has been deemed unacceptable and has thus become an increasingly pervasive notion for human existence in western societies. Risk is a central aspect of human subjectivity, seen as something that has to be managed through human intervention, and it is associated with notions of choice, responsibility and blame (Lupton, 1999). In advanced industrial societies, a "risk society" is one in which the notion of the subject is dissolved and replaced with "factors of risk" (Castel, 1991), and where administering the health of populations through new technologies of care (e.g., health promotion) has become paramount (Castel, 1991; Lupton, 1995; Rose, 2007).

Risk has thus become a defining feature of modern society and pervades all aspects of everyday life, filling it with perceived physical, moral, psychological, social, technological, economic, geopolitical and environmental dangers (Lester & Russell, 2014). The science of risk calculation, assessment and evaluation has become the hallmark of modernity's progress by rationalisation and calculation, "from the actuarial tables of life insurers to the risk analysis of those in the business of risk: the movers and shakers of capitalism" (Fox, 1999 cited in Lester & Russell, 2014, p. 1). The technology of risk-assessment is entangled with knowledge, instruments, bodies, institutions and spaces to form assumptions about life and to shape patterns of governance. The drive to minimise risks to human health extends, for example, to the reduction of injury and the nurturing of children.

A key feature of what is called the "biopolitics of risk" is the governing of human conduct; people are placed under constant surveillance while at the same time are increasingly encouraged to monitor themselves (i.e., parents monitoring their children's behaviour and children monitoring themselves and their active play) (Wright & Harwood, 2009). It marks a political and ethical field where individuals are obliged to assess and make responsible choices with the intention of minimising exposure to health hazards. Failure to do so labels individuals as "risky", generating both societal disapproval and also potentially feelings of personal shame, despair or disengagement. Rose (1999) calls this the "responsibilization of life", and Beck (1992) refers to it as "individualisation", in which more and more aspects of behaviour are subject to self-reflection and self-management. Evaluating risk establishes a moral dimension to bodily behaviour, creating a hierarchy between those who choose to use the advice in "safe" ways to manage their bodies, and those who do not.

This modern conception of risk inevitably contributes to the formation of childhood, marking it as a period during the life-course in which the child needs protecting from the multiple risks that lie in wait to cause harm. Perceived contemporary social ills have increasingly threatened this state of "innocence" and have produced ever-increasing levels of risk-anxiety for parents. As such, the child has become the target of social, political, educational and legal regulations that constitute children as the powerless and dependent (Ryall, Russell, & MacLean, 2013).

Thus, the discourse of risk has material consequences that are played out and negotiated in everyday relationships and spaces: parental anxieties and responsibilities have delimited children's ability to negotiate time/space away from adults, while childcare workers and teachers are guarded in their contact with children. Health and education institutions have co-emerged as central pillars in this project and have increasingly spread their regimes and accounting procedures into other sectors. Of particular relevance to this chapter is that children's play has become caught up in this biopolitical, technical yet redemptive project. The following sections of this chapter consider how play has become entangled in the material discursive practices of risk, health and well-being (Lester & Russell, 2014).

Finally, the historical movement of children playing freely in diverse spaces to children playing in designated play spaces (playgrounds, school gymnasiums, sports fields, recreation centres and friends' houses) has been socially and culturally underpinned by a "culture of fear" around childhood generally. Risk narratives have discursively circulated around risk and children's independent mobility, risk in playgrounds, risk and responsibility and finally, the risk in *not* playing. These are related to general concerns about children's free time (Aitken, 2001; Holloway & Valentine, 2000) and parental safety concerns (Valentine, 2004), specifically the dangers of the urban built environment and its corollaries (i.e., increased traffic, stranger-danger, bullying) (Mitra, Faulkner, Buliung, & Stone, 2014). We draw on a selection of children's narratives to illustrate children's perspectives on risky play and their attempts to freely range beyond the confines of home to develop their own play landscapes. We then turn our attention towards calls for children to engage in outdoor and risky play again, and we examine the growing institutional, community and media narratives and academic literatures that are part of that movement.

Children's movement and mobility

Where did risk discourses about play emerge? In the last 150 years, as we have illustrated in the preceding chapters, there have been many shifts in how children, parents, public health agencies, children's societies and educationalists have regarded the issue of play and the risks involved if children do not play "properly". These shifts have corresponded with ideologies around childhood, parenting, poverty, immigration, urban development, education and citizenship, to name but a few. While these shifts were not universal for children, and affected children differently in different times and in different places, what is noticeable is a historical, social and cultural trajectory to remove children from playing outside in the streets and engaging in a diverse range of activities into demarcated and spatially bound areas. These areas included playgrounds and school gymnasiums, but also subsequently, a move to spatially specific organised sports and house-bound forms of play, such as "play dates" (Frost, 2010).

However, after decades of containing children's activities and attempting to reduce the risks in play, there is now a new focus on encouraging their ability to navigate streets, get outside and practice their independence. Indeed, a term is now used for children's independent movement outdoors: children's independent mobility (CIM) (Schoeppe, Duncan, Badland, Oliver, & Curtis, 2013; Crawford et al., 2017). CIM refers to children's ability to move around in public spaces without adult accompaniment and includes, among other things, active modes of transportation and independent free play. According to Carver, Veitch, Sahlqvist, Crawford, and Hume (2014), in Australia, children "roam" little, with only one-third of 8–15 year old children who are permitted to venture alone more than 15 minutes from their homes. Similarly, in a newspaper article entitled "How children lost the right to roam in four generations in England", Derbyshire (2007) highlights the erosion of children's capacity to roam over four generations, and he includes a map depicting the containment of children's movement from the early 1900s until 2007 (see Figure 5.2). He cites a report published by *Natural England* and the *Royal Society for the Protection of Birds* that "warns that the mental health of 21st-century children is at risk because they are missing out on the exposure to the natural world enjoyed by past generations" (p. 1).

A more recent report from 2015 (*State of Play Survey*) published by the *Human Potential Centre* in New Zealand indicated that less than half of children aged 8–12 in New Zealand are allowed to travel alone in their neighbourhood, with only around 5% doing so frequently (Human Potential Centre, 2015). This, despite their parents recalling weekends spent riding their bikes to friends' houses, exploring the local bush or walking alone to the nearest shopping malls.

Concurrent with the rise of car culture, the development of "dangerous" urban sprawl, parental fears about the dangers of living in urban areas and the growing density of inner cities in many western industrialised nations, there is also now the fear of living in obesogenic environments (Carroll-Scott et al., 2013) as fewer and fewer natural (green) spaces are available for play (IPA, 2016). This, in combination with media stories about child abductions and societal dangers (Lindon, 1999; Landry, 2005), increasing perceptions of "stranger-danger", violence and bullying (Valentine, 2004), the presence of "weirdos" in one's neighbourhood (Crawford et al., 2017) or fears over environmental pollutants (Taylor, Pollard, Angus, & Rocks, 2013) have had a sustained influence on children's play and outdoor life

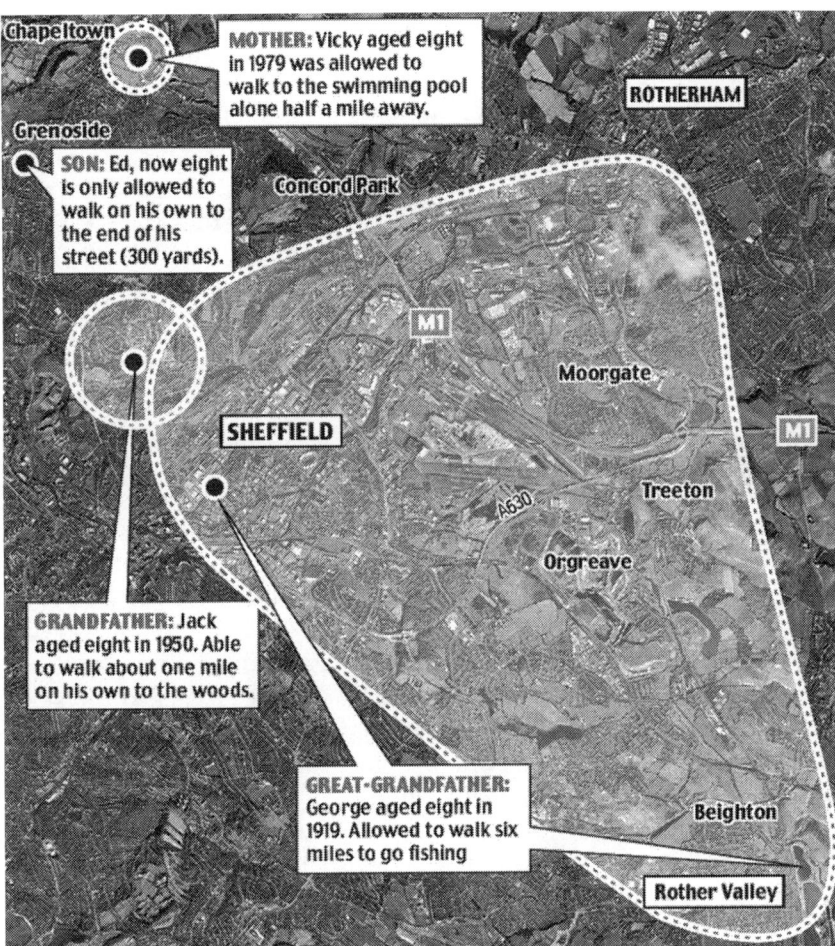

Figure 5.2 "How children lost the right to roam in four generations in England" (Daily Mail Online).

Source: "How children lost the right to roam in four generations" (2007), David Derbyshire. Reprinted with permission.

(Buliung, Mitra, & Faulkner, 2009; Stone, Faulkner, Mitra, & Buliung, 2014; Wheway & Millwar, 1997). Consequently, this has created physical, social and cultural environments that exacerbate parental fears about children's unsupervised outdoor play. Partly resulting from these augmented fears regarding CIM, research by the *Future Foundations* (2006) found that the time children spend in adult care had quadrupled between

1975 and 2001, which was largely because parents were growing evermore fearful of leaving their children unsupervised – this of course has implications for children's spontaneous free play in public and outdoor spaces (Thompson, Travlou, & Roe, 2006).

In a study of parental perceptions of play in England, Valentine and McKendrick (1997) found that the greatest influence on children's independent play appeared to be parental anxieties about safety and what they call the "changing nature of childhood". They suggest that there were:

> moral panics about everything from child murderers and teenage gangs, to joy riding and juvenile crime rates . . . fears that public space is being overrun by violent and unruly teenagers who are a threat to the personal safety of young children.
>
> (p. 223)

The authors argue that overall, whether playing independently outdoors in the garden, or even at institutionally based play activities, children are simply spending more time under adult supervision (Valentine & McKendrick, 1997). A similar study in Australia (Crawford et al., 2017), found that parents' safety concerns about CIM fell into two broad categories: risks posed by people and traffic-related risks. Parents were concerned that their children might get lost or that they lacked the skills required for safely negotiating traffic, and recognising and responding to risks. There was a sense that their children were not ready to confront the risks that urban environments entailed. Furthermore, parents took cues from other parents, schools, the media and perceived community norms with regard to what was acceptable behaviour with regard to CIM, both on the part of the children and the parents. While parents felt that other parents judged them, they also passed judgement easily on the decisions of others, particularly with regard to those who allowed their children what was considered "too much" freedom.

Concrete recent examples of this have involved police and child protection services in the United States: in 2015 a Montgomery County family was accused of neglect because they let their children walk alone to school (twice) (St. George, 2015), and in December 2014, local police enforcement and *Child Protective Services* were called in when a brother and sister, aged 10 and 6, were walking a mile along a six-lane avenue just north of Washington, D.C. (Griffin, 2015). However, concerns about risk, though perhaps most frequent, are not only relevant to the USA. As Frost (2010) notes "the culture of fear is increasing and paranoid parenting is making rapid inroads into childhood culture in the UK" (p. 226).

Playgrounds: design and safety

One of the most important areas of risk incursion on children's play has involved playground equipment and activities. Indeed, playground design has increasingly focused on child safety, but as a consequence of this safety focus, playgrounds became less about play and have been rendered less interesting and somewhat sterile (Brunelle, Coghlan, Herrington, & Brussoni, 2016; Veitch, Bagley, Ball, & Salmon, 2006). In Canada, the technical standards for the physical features of children's outdoor play spaces are provided by the *Canadian Standards Association (CSA)* (Herrington & Nicholls, 2007). The idea to expand the CSA's area of expertise from objects such as mechanical refrigeration and gas equipment standards (its original mandate) to children's outdoor play spaces was hatched in 1979 when the *Canadian Institute of Child Health* and the *Canadian Council of Social Development* conducted an informal investigation of playground injuries entitled *Danger: Children at Play!* Unfortunately, when this task force lobbied for the establishment of standards addressing outdoor play spaces they ignored Canadian studies suggesting that injury levels on playgrounds were not significantly high. This resulted in the inflation of perceived risk in a Canadian context, further inciting fear about the risks involved in outdoor play spaces. As such, a culture of fear was cultivated with regard to children's playgrounds, with risk avoidance dominating. Furthermore, these fears are exacerbated by media headlines such as "Playground equipment involved in rising number of injuries: Experts concerned about lack of mandatory standards" published by the *Canadian Broadcasting Corporation (CBC)* (2013). The article reports that:

> More than 28,000 children are injured every year on playgrounds across Canada, and the rate of hospitalizations has gone up by eight per cent between 2007 and 2012, CBC News has learned. Even though playgrounds continue to be upgraded and made safer, experts point to a lack of consistent standards – together with problems maintaining playground surfaces properly – with the continuing rate of injury. In all jurisdictions in Canada, play structures only need to adhere to the *Canadian Standards Association* standards in the year they were built, and no upgrades are mandatory. Some experts think that has to change.
>
> (CBC, 2013, p. 1)

The article cited experts who stated that about 10% of children who do get hospitalised from playground injuries require many interventions including surgeries and rehabilitation. Indeed, many experts advocate for a ban on play structures that are not approved by the CSA. While there are some who profit from the fear that there are "dangers lurking in playgrounds and parks" (see www.personalinjurylawyerservice.ca/articles-playground-dangers), there is in fact much more acceptance and encouragement of playgrounds that provide risker forms of play (Boesveld, 2012; Osler, 2016). The problem with the CSA's historical breadth of influence in policy development for children's play spaces stems from the fact that the standards focus on technical information concerning structural integrity, performance requirements and the maintenance of materials and play structures, leaving out the needs and desires of children. However, advocates such as the *International School Grounds Alliance (ISGA)*, whose members hail from Australia, Canada, Germany, Japan, Sweden, the United Kingdom and the United States, seek to address the "increasingly sedentary and risk-averse generation of children disconnected from nature" and they hope to "become an influential force that will help schools see the learning opportunities that can come from peering under rocks and maybe even skinning a knee during recess" (Boesveld, 2012, p. 1). As Boesveld (2012) cites:

> "We're not fans of broken arms", said Cam Collyer, co-founder of the ISGA and program director of *Evergreen Canada*, a national charity that promotes healthy communities. "But we're fans of broken arms if there's enormous play and learning value on a landscape instead of providing a flat barren space."
>
> (p. 1)

Indeed, the counter-movement to make playgrounds "riskier" in Canada has led the Canadian non-profit *Lawson Foundation* to recently announce $2.7 million in grant money for 18 Canadian projects as part of its outdoor play strategy. The funds are to develop play spaces not "where kids can get seriously injured, but rather spaces that encourage more calculated risks" (Osler, 2016, p. 1). Increasingly one can read headlines in newspapers where adults are now asking, "has old-fashioned fun been trumped by fears of injury and legal action?" (CBC, 2016, p. 1).

In alignment with this, in our study, when children discussed their play activities, some voiced frustration at the dominance of risk-aversion in their school grounds. For example, Arman a 9-year-old boy talked about the restrictions imposed on how he would like to play in his school playground:

A: The teachers don't like it when your head is hanging down. They don't like it when it's like that . . . they find it dangerous.
INTERVIEWER: And you?
A: It's cool. It's not dangerous, it's cool.
INTERVIEWER: Why is it cool?
A: Because when you're hanging upside down you can make more figures than when you are upright . . . I can hang upside down for hours and hours . . . it's forbidden.

Indeed, risk avoidance in school grounds has not focused on playground equipment alone. For instance, in a recent article from the *San Francisco Chronicle* (Tucker, 2017), cited at the beginning of this chapter, the journalist describes a school in Alameda County, California where tag, along with a litany of other games have been banned due to safety concerns. The general rule for recess at this school is based on three questions: "Is it safe? Is it kind? Is it responsible?" (p. 1). Nowhere is fun mentioned. Similarly, "No Ball Playing" by-laws, which corresponded with developing suburban sprawl, were linked to the development of a litigious society with respect to children's play (Frost, 2010). Suburban sprawl saw the eradication of sidewalks and house-front green spaces to facilitate parking and easier commuter traffic (Moore, 1987). In Canada, increasing bureaucracy, risk and lawsuit fears resulted in silencing the scurrying of sticks (i.e., hockey sticks) on many side-streets in major cities. One newspaper outlet concluded:

> While once-fit children slowly gained weight and found other pastimes, like smoking weed and joining gangs, the city plastered its glaring white notices, Ball and Hockey Playing *Prohibited*, citing by-law 522–78.
> (City News Staff, 2016, p. 1)

In July 2016, after almost 40 years, the ban on playing street hockey and basketball was lifted in Canada's largest metropolitan city – Toronto. While there are some who still disagree with playing in the streets because it may put children at risk, and the city may be liable for injury and safety, many, including the Mayor of Toronto and the *Provincial Ontario Children and Youth Services* urged Toronto city council to lift the ban (Benzie, 2016). Many of the calls to lift the ban were aligned with some of the public health discourses we alluded to earlier in the book around childhood obesity rates and concerns about children's levels of (in)activity. Notably, notions of nostalgia, pleasure and play are raised, such as in a statement made recently by a Toronto City Councillor:

> Most of us grew up playing hockey in the streets. . . . It's something that most of us have grown up playing and it's part of the fabric of Canada.
> (Mehta, 2016, p. 1)

These kinds of comments are not unlike the language used in the *Canadian Tire* advertisements *We all play for Canada*, one of which was discussed in Chapter 3. While drawing on the mythical relationship between hockey and Canadian pride, connections are made between a Canadian pastime, health, obesity and taking risks through outdoor street play.

One might conclude, drawing on the words of Castel (1991), that all this "grandiose technocratic rationalizing dream of absolute control of the accidental, understood as the irruption of the unpredictable" (p. 289) has been well cultivated with regard to the organisation and regulation of play(grounds). Specifically, such discourses on risk are directed at the regulation of the body – in this case the child's body – and "how it moves in space, how it interacts with other bodies and things" (Lupton, 1999 p. 88). In risk-aversion societies, then, particularly when children and their play activities are involved (Gill, 2007), play and play spaces, as we noted previously, are often subjected to multiple risk assessments, which can diminish the excitement and pleasure for children (Gleave, 2008; Jachyra & Fusco, 2016). Moreover, it justifies adult interventions to minimise risk, and maximise the productivity of their bodies (Foucault, 1991; Dean, 1999; Lupton, 1999).

The psychologist Peter Gray (2011) has argued that there is a direct link between generational increases in psychopathology and declines in play-time and children's agentic opportunities. Thus, the reproduction of standardised, homogeneous playgrounds and concerns about playground safety (Ball, 2002; Franklin, 2002; Frost, 2010), as well as the growth of a litigious society, or what Gill (2007) labels a "compensation culture", have all led to an era of play deprivation and a reduction in play value and risk-taking for children, whose effects we have not quite realised (Frost, 2010). Despite the overwhelming desires to allow children the freedom to roam, to develop resourcefulness and exhibit their agentic capacities (Lester & Russell, 2008) and public health's call to move children outside and take some risks, there may be lingering fears about children's outdoor play and independent mobility (Faulkner, Mitra, Buliung, Fusco, & Stone, 2015), especially for those marginalised by gender, class, ability and race/ethnicity (Lindon, 1999; Morrongiello & Dawber, 1998). However, what we are seeing now is that public health and other health and physical activity organisations are taking a leading role in promoting a new set of discourses about risky outdoor and free play. With questions such as "Want to get active? Just get outside!" (See ParticipACTION, 2016a), and policies such as *No Freedom to Roam* (Active Healthy Kids England, 2016), *Getting it Right for Play* (Play Scotland, 2017) and the *No Child Left Inside Act* (Louv, 2008), public health and physical activity organisations are seizing the opportunity to be the arbiter of how risk-taking and play should be understood, what kinds of play are useful and worthwhile, and which are not. It seems that today a lot still rests on play.

Responsibility and the regulation of risk

Institutional control of risk

With the advent of compulsory schooling in various western industrialised nations in the 19th and 20th centuries, adults' fears about the risks and dangers of unsupervised and unlimited playing could be mitigated because children could now be contained in surveyed and controlled educational and play/physical activity spaces. Historically, the movement of play into schools and playgrounds, which had the benefit of addressing child pauperism, illiteracy and "useless" activity, had the spin-off effect of reducing risk as it led to the development of more disciplined activities for children across all social classes (Frost, 2010; Kirk, 1998, 2001). From a public health perspective, corralling children in schools, where they could now be subjected to normative policies around hygiene and health (Foucault, 1978), served as a means for reducing risks of disease. This focus aligned with the emergence of what Foucault (1978) has called a "biopolitics of population" which was ultimately linked to the management and administration of life, normativity and nationhood.

Under this kind of regime of population government, not surprisingly, play and independent mobility for children, as we have noted, gave way to physical drills, which focused on regulation and organisation (Kirk, 1998). The transformation of play into exercise left few places for imagination, pleasure or risk-taking. Instead play became more calculated as it served the ever-increasing focus on militarisation and the character-building sports/play ethos of modern sport and physical education (Mangan, 1981). Indeed, the history of physical education globally and specifically in the USA (Zeigler, 1979), England (McIntosh, 1968), Canada (Cosentino & Howell, 1971) and Australia (Kirk, 1998) from the mid-1800s to the 1920s shows how play and risk-taking in play (e.g., children getting dirty, falling, exploring areas on their own) became increasingly subservient to the emphasis on controlled drill exercises. A commitment to these new educational and national paradigms meant containing risk and moving towards more "specialised means of schooling bodies" (Kirk, 2001, p. 475). Bringing together physical training, sport and health inspections meant increasing surveillance, regulation and rationalisation of children's (play) activities in ways that would not only allow for adult control over children's free time, but also had the beneficial effect of developing strong and young bodies to service the nation (Kirk, 2001).

With the rise of the Cold War (1950s onwards), the increases in consumer societies, the growth of car culture and the development of suburbs – all things that spawned an anxiousness over the decline of national fitness – children's imaginative and free play was curbed more and more. Rather than free, unstructured play in which children learned by taking risks, prescribed physical activity was politically, socially and culturally sanctioned as new discourses of health and the medicalisation of society became pervasive (Foucault, 1980; Rose, 2007). Subsequently, national fitness took hold in the 1950s–1960s, as did the means to achieve it, through scientifically determined physical education programmes (Evans, Davies, & Wright, 2004), organised youth sports in the USA, Britain, Canada, Australia and New Zealand (Gatz, Messner, & Ball-Rokeach, 2002; Kremer, Trew, & Ogle, 1997) and an (re)emphasis on early child development through play in contained spaces (Frost, 2005). All of these practices aligned with new sociocultural beliefs about risk-aversion (Beck, 1992). As we mentioned in chapter 3, some of the children in our study felt constrained by sports activities, and felt 'freer' engaging in play that was more self-directed. It could be argued that through the institutional control of risk, children have been robbed of their agentic capacity, while the *techne* of sports and fitness has come to dominate the *poesies* of play (Heidegger, 1954 in Pronger, 2002, p. 58).

Parental control of risk

Historically, the increasing numbers of children entering organised sports gave rise to another phenomenon that further contained children's independent mobility – "the mother taxi" (Thompson, 1999). Instead of children finding their own way to their events, parents, particularly mothers, were charged with mitigating the risk of independent movement by driving their children and other people's children to and from games/sports. While children were active playing their sports, they now lost the opportunity to walk, bike, skateboard or take a scooter to their sports events, which further reduced their playful opportunities. This is a phenomenon that has not been lost on those in public health concerned with the reduction in children's active transportation opportunities (Buliung et al., 2009; Veitch et al., 2017). An exploration of the often polarising contemporary discussions around play and whether children have access to outdoor play highlights the role of the parents as a central factor in determining the safety of their child's activities (Ball, 2004; Ball, Gill, & Spiegal, 2008; Boufous, Finch, & Bauman, 2004; Brussoni, Olsen, Pike, & Sleet, 2012; Carver, Timperio, & Crawford, 2008; Sandseter, 2009a; Sandseter & Kennair, 2011; Timperio, Crawford, Telford, & Salmon, 2004; Valentine & McKendrick, 1997; Veitch et al., 2006). Recent literature suggests that in neo-liberal times the family has been thoroughly pedagogised (Burrows, 2016; Dagkas & Quarmby, 2012; Fullagar, 2009). As the target of government interventions, the family is increasingly becoming "an important site for the transmission of knowledge and cultural values" around physical activity (Dagkas & Burrows, 2016, p. 1). Indeed, Dagkas and Burrows argue that governmental resources and interventions "are premised on and indeed rely on parental anxiety, fear, risk, guilt and 'love'" (p. 6). They continue:

> parents, their investments in their children, their anxieties about what they may become and their guilt if failing to provide the requisite resources to fulfil their potential are needed to "make things work". On the one hand ... parents are oft-times regarded as obstacles to health and physical activity work; on the other, their commitment to the products and services conveyed is seemingly pivotal to the success of health and physical activity initiatives.
>
> (p. 6)

Mothers, specifically, are often blamed for their children's welfare (Ladd-Taylor & Umansky, 1998; Jackson & Mannix, 2004). Maternal responsibilisation (Parker, 2014), which focuses on the responsibility of mothers for their own health and their child's health and behaviour, is also increasingly apparent in Canadian narratives about changes to children's play. For example, ParticipACTION's (2011) *Think Again* campaign targets mothers as responsible for making sure their children are active enough. In one of the campaign's advertisements, a mother considers her child's physical activity, saying to the audience, "My Jamie plays soccer twice a week, that's plenty of activity!" Suddenly, a soccer ball appears from the sidelines and hits her on the shoulder. The words "Think again" in bold cross the screen, and the next image reads: "Fact is, kids need at least 60 minutes of physical activity per day. Every day".

Another advertisement from the same campaign depicts a mother saying that her child swims a few times a week, the mother figure is then doused with water before the screen is similarly emblazoned with the words *Think Again* and a warning that more physical activity is needed for children. While there have been evaluations of the *Think Again* campaign and its effectiveness in encouraging parents generally (Gainforth et al., 2015), and mothers specifically (Berry et al., 2014), to increase their children's physical activity levels, these articles have failed to critique the responsibilisation placed on mothers. Mother-blame is particularly insidious. First, it normalises gender roles in society (i.e., mothers as primary caretakers of their children). Second, although women are perceived as engaging in less risk (Lupton, 1999), implicitly, mothers are held responsible for putting their children at risk for physical inactivity and for lacking in the knowledge required for raising healthy physically active children (Boero, 2009; Friedman, 2014; Parker, 2014; McNaughton, 2011).

Additionally, there is now an emerging critique against parents for "helicopter parenting" or "over-parenting". Mostly, in popular culture, and aligning with public health advocacy organisations, there are calls for parents to "not stand between your kids and the great outdoors" (ParticipACTION, 2015) and to let children engage with risk. For years parents (especially mothers) have been told to control their children's risk-taking and yet now parents (again, especially mothers) are being told to allow their children – even encourage them – to take risks. Parents (most often mothers) are now criticised for over-parenting and for not giving their children more play opportunities and freedom (Tremblay et al., 2015; Veitch et al., 2006). Indeed, public health agencies, which have for years focused on minimising risks in children's play, have learned from the critiques of risk-prevention or aversion and have begun to embrace a new era of risk promotion. However, as more and more responsibility for play and its risk management is placed on parents, responsibility is removed from the municipal, provincial/state/county and federal governments to provide for livable and playable environments for their citizens, as well as opportunities for healthy risk-taking in play. As Lupton (1996) suggests, in the context of neo-liberal economics, governments want the benefits of an active, healthy citizenry and extol the virtues of a "participatory imperative" (Lupton, 1996), which places the responsibility for safety, health and well-being solely on individual citizens (Crawford, 1980; Ingham, 1985; Petersen & Lupton, 1996; Wheway, 2008).

Taking risks (or any intimation of danger) with respect to play has historically and culturally been avoided at all cost, especially by parents. Children's physical safety (i.e., an absence of all physical harm) has been of foremost importance. As such, for many families with young children, it seems perhaps subversive, even irresponsible and legally questionable to conceive of encouraging one's children to play in a way in which physical risk might be possible (Alexander et al., 2015; Cooper, 2000). Marianne, a 10-year-old girl in our study, was cognizant of parental risk control.

> Well, in our back alley sometimes, the kids playing are not supervised, and sometimes there are parents who come and ask us: "have you seen my child? I don't see him anymore?" So, then it's like, "you should supervise your child, it's dangerous!" At the park, well, I can't go alone . . . I'm not allowed. And when we're in the alley, well, anything can happen, so my mom says she always has to be in the yard to supervise me. And, when we are in the yard, she has to be somewhere close by where she can supervise us in the yard.

Parents are therefore in somewhat of a bind – they can be vilified if they allow their children to take risks, but since hyper-parenting is also associated with reduced physical activity (Janssen, 2015) and other negative effects (LeMoyne & Buchanan, 2011), they are also made responsible for exposing their children to a new set of risks with respect to physical (in)activity and sedentariness (Boulos, Kuross Vikre, Oppenheimer, Chang, & Kanarek, 2012). And, as Dagkas and Burrows (2016) argue, how parents are perceived affects the way children are addressed for their physical activities:

> From helicopter varieties to recalcitrant parents and those whom teachers envisage as simply ill-equipped to provide children with the resources they need to develop healthy habits, it is clear that how parents are thought about, what they are assumed to bring (or not) to their offsprings' well-being matters. It shapes how family pedagogues think about their students/clients/recipients of health messages and it informs how they envisage their role in health and/or physical activity promotion.
>
> (p. 6)

Not playing outside is not optional

The AHKC and ParticipACTION *Physical Activity Report Cards* developed and made popular in Canada (described in previous chapters) have now been reproduced by organisations around the world (see *Active Healthy Kids England Report Card*, 2016; *Active Healthy Kids Scotland Report Card*, 2016, and *Active Healthy Kids Australia Report Card*, 2016). As mentioned previously, there is now an international consortium of 38 countries that release report cards on children's physical (in)activity (see Active Health Kids Global Alliance, 2017). The global groups producing the report cards suggest that combatting decreasing physical activity rates requires an increased acceptance of risk for physical activity promotion. In Canada, there is also now increasing concern that being indoors is both preventing physical activity, and opening children up to the risks of online bullying, harassment and breathing stagnant indoor air (ParticipACTION, 2017). As we noted previously in Chapter 3, popular campaigns such as the *Canadian Tire* advertisement emphasise a world outside that awaits children – lonely sports equipment waits for two eager hands, swings wait for children to swing, and fields and forests wait to be discovered, if only adults would let their children roam freely and leaving them to play "until the streetlights are turned on" (Canadian Tire, 2013).

In a recent newspaper interview for the *Ottawa Sun* in 2017, Mark Tremblay (Director of the *Healthy Active Living and Obesity Research Group*, HALO, at the *Children's Hospital of Eastern Ontario Research Institute*) decries the fact that contemporary children's physical activity and play is less mobile and less risky than in previous eras. A segment of this interview explains:

> According to Tremblay's report, the waist circumference of a 12-year-old girl increased by six centimetres in the 1981/2007 comparison. The grip strength of a boy declined by 10 per cent. As Tremblay says, these findings make sense when we imagine the cultural shift in childhood activities over the past 30 years. Children were outside every free moment, climbing trees, throwing balls and wrestling after school. They gripped sticks and fired snowballs. "Just thinking about grip strength, children today grip, very gently, their smart phone, not a tree branch, and not the scruff of someone's neck," says Tremblay. At 55, he grew up playing outside, as did most of his generation. . . . A culture change is required, as fundamental as a glance back to Canada's past, a simpler time when we spent hours outside engaged in work and play. Those same electronic devices holding adults and children in a spell deliver overwrought tales from around the globe of danger lurking around the corner. "If you send your eight-year-old out to play on his own some nosy neighbour is going to call child services and a whole orchestration is involved," Tremblay says. In the 1960s if a child wasn't outside playing, neighbours would have thought that family strange. Fear permeates our culture, and not just because of the latest terrorist attack. Dr. Tremblay notes dryly, "you can't go out in the morning because of mosquitoes and the risk of West Nile (virus)". Later in the day, there is rush hour

traffic . . . pollution. Sun causes skin cancer. "So, you can't go out at any point in time." The solution seems simple. Shake the fear and open the door. Instantly, activity levels rise, sedentary behaviours wane. . . . "It's there. It's free. I can go there right now and do something and so can everyone." . . . "As we reflect back on 150 years, we have a heritage as frontiers people – nature and the outdoors are almost synonymous with what it was like to be Canadian, whether it's canoeing across a lake or snowshoeing through a forest," Tremblay says. "And the great outdoors is still there. We are the second biggest country in the world, probably the most beautiful, and physical activity opportunities are endless."

(Scanlan, 2017, p. 1)

Simultaneously, the outdoors is constituted as free, natural, essential for children's physically active play, and is constituted as having acceptable levels of risk (ParticipACTION, 2016b). In its recent *Position Statement on Active Outdoor Play*, ParticipACTION (2016b) extols the virtues of allowing children access to active play in nature and the outdoors with all its corresponding risks:

> Risk is seen as a bad word . . . But in play, risk doesn't mean courting danger – like skating on a half-frozen pond or sending a preschooler to the park alone. It means the types of play children see as thrilling and exciting, where the possibility of physical injury may exist, but they can recognize and evaluate the challenges according to their own ability. It means giving children the freedom to decide how high to climb, to explore the woods, get dirty, play hide 'n seek, wander in their neighbourhoods, balance, tumble and rough-house, especially outdoors.
>
> (p. 1)

Whereas before children were dissuaded from engaging in risky activities (i.e., extreme or counter-culture sports, cycling and walking on busy streets), now simply being indoors with access to screens and breathing indoor air is deemed risky, and is blamed for childhood inactivity and increases in chronic health conditions. Indeed, socio-cultural adherences to risk-aversion, while having improved child protection, safety guidelines and harm reduction, are now made responsible for the demise of active outdoor play (Tremblay et al., 2015). Risky play has been reconstituted as "thrilling and exciting play that can include the possibility of physical injury" such as "play at height, speed, near dangerous elements . . . where there is potential for disappearing or getting lost" (Tremblay et al.,

2015, p. 5). While the *Position Statement* is not a "how to" document for increasing risky outdoor play, the authors suggest:

> it was designed to be a foundation of credible evidence from which programs, strategies, campaigns, policies, practices and environmental modifications [for outdoor play] can be provoked, initiated and supported.
>
> (Tremblay et al., 2015, p. 8)

The *Position Statement* thus provides physiological, social, epidemiological and behavioural evidence to demonstrate that risky outdoor play facilitates healthy and active development. The authors argue that a shift in perceptions of socio-cultural risk is necessary in order to move away from and beyond perspectives of danger and towards new ideas about challenge, adventure and opportunity concluding that there is a strong relationship between outdoor play and children's health (Brussoni et al., 2015; Gray et al., 2015).

Amidst the competing and contradictory discourses and debates about risk (e.g., risks outdoors, risks indoors, promoting children's risky play), about playground safety (see Ball, 2002), and the contributing factors to perceptions of risk (e.g., age, socialisation, parenting style, socio-cultural environment) (Morrongiello & Lasenby-Lessard, 2007), there have been sustained calls by communities and public policy-makers in Canada, USA, UK, Australia and New Zealand that align with ParticipACTION's *Position Statement* (2016b) to encourage children to "take back the streets" (Playing Out, 2017), (re)discover their "wildhoods" (Go RVing Canada, 2017) and to get back to nature (ParticipACTION, 2016b). Indeed, numerous play researchers and risk advocates argue for the necessity to include risk in children's lives – particularly in outdoor play – but do not start with concerns about obesity or physical inactivity as their departure point. Instead they argue that taking risks in play activities builds character. As a counter-response to a socio-cultural fear of risk, a group of play scholars and advocates have conducted research on the possible benefits of risk and risk-taking in play for children (Gill, 2007, 2009, 2010; Sandseter, 2009a, 2009b; Sandseter & Kennair, 2011). For instance, Gill (2010), an advocate for risk-in-play, argues that historically and culturally, anxiety over children's safety has led adults to underestimate children's abilities. Such anxieties have limited children's "very experiences that help them to learn how to handle the challenges that life may throw at them" (p. 1). Others have written about the benefits of risks and about the enjoyment children feel when engaging in and mastering a particular risk. Sandseter (2009b) studied the characteristics of risky play in a Norwegian context and has examined why children engage in risky play.

She writes that children enjoy risky play for the "excitement and the joy of mastering a risky and potentially dangerous situation" (p. 7); it was through explorative and risky play that children familiarised themselves with their environment, "its possibilities and boundaries" (p. 7), and learned to judge what is a danger and how to manage it (Alexander et al., 2015). In our study, Alain, a 9-year-old boy described how he learned to master a risky manoeuvre on his bike.

A: So, you have the bike here and you have a bar that holds your seat [cross bar]. Well, I put my feet on that bar . . . and then I stand up, except that I'm still holding the handle bars.
I: So you're standing on your bike?
A: Ya, because I'm going really fast, and I don't fall because I hold on pretty well. I'm also kind of used to it. . . . It took a long time before I knew how to do it. Before, I used to just put my feet on the bar, and I was afraid of standing up. Then I stood up a little. Then I got used to it, so I did the big standing figure.
I: Who taught you to do that?
A: No one, I learned it on my own.

There is now a growing academic literature and government policies devoted to increasing environmental and natural experiences for children and young people (Gill, 2014; Muñoz, 2009), and for creating and producing built environments that are child-friendly (Hart, 2003). There are also very well-established discourses, policies and practices directed towards children's "right to play" (International Play Association, 2016) and a growing movement on the child's right to the city (Bartlett, 2002; Hart, 2002; Riggio, 2002; Yates, 2003). Urban and city planners, politicians, child advocates and researchers from across disciplinary areas (e.g., sociology, geography, education, childhood studies, epidemiologists etc.) argue that "children's well-being is shaped by where they live" and that "the quality of play is fundamentally shaped by the environment where it happens" (International Play Association, 2016, p. 1). These calls for child-friendly cities and risk-free environments – ones that promote play – *are not aligned* with the biopolitical regimes that discursively produce children's physical (in)activity as an "epidemic" (Petherick, 2015; Rail, 2012; Rich, 2010b; Rich & Evans, 2009), but are rather about providing children with the right to "engage in spontaneous play, recreation and creativity" (International Play Association, 2017, p. 1). This is an important contradistinction to public health's claims for children's play as a means to fitness.

Lastly, these varied discussions of risk have emerged at the same time as the growing movement around "free-range parenting", which is based on the popularised notion that children deserve some unsupervised time. Griffin (2015) writes:

> The goals of a free-range parent are the same as those of most parents: to raise their kids to cope successfully with life, and if possible, be outrageously happy. Humans have been debating how to get your kid to be a successful adult since we began to speak. For free-range parents, the answer is autonomy and responsibility – early and often.
> (p. 1)

The "free range parenting" movement has been controversial, and as Zamosky (2009) writes, it has also received some sensational media attention:

> Would you let your 9-year-old son ride the New York City Subway system alone? Columnist Lenore Skenazy did, and then she wrote about the experience in the New York Sun. What followed was a storm of media attention and a mix of accolades and accusations from parents everywhere. A new movement also grew from Skenazy's bold move: It's called free-range parenting.
> (p. 1)

Lenore Skenazy (2017), who stated that she has been dubbed "America's worst mom" (p. 1), has trademarked the term *FreeRangeKids* as a "commonsense approach to parenting in these overprotective times" (Skenazy, 2017, p. 1). She writes:

> We're swimming in fear soup – fear of lawsuits, fear of injury, fear of abductions, fear of blame. (People love to blame parents for not being "responsible" enough.) And Free-Range Kids is trying to paddle out.
> (p. 2)

The backlash from free-range parenting movements and from public health advocacy groups against an overprotective risk society and against the systemic fear of the outdoors aligns with what we are arguing here – that fear of risk may indeed cause problems for how parents and children negotiate their independent movement. This has implications for children's play and well-being and also for the responsibilisation of parents. What we find potentially problematic is that this now increasing encouragement for children to take risks in play may simply become another prescription or requirement that parents and children have to consider. So, while risk-taking viewed as beneficial for play, it is important to re-emphasise, it may bring with it more judgement and responsibility (Burrows, 2009) and more surveillance (Rich, 2010a) for those parents and children who fail to take up these new prescriptions. As Dagkas and Burrows (2016) argue:

> Rendered variously responsible for the ill health of children and capable of ameliorating it, the interest in families as sites for health surveillance, monitoring, enhancement, sport participation, and as hubs for fostering physical fitness has burgeoned. Imperatives such as "families need to . . ." and "families should . . ." pepper healthy and physical activity policies.
>
> (p. 1)

Conclusion

Studies in the UK and New Zealand demonstrate that many children seek out risk-taking play activities (Gill, 2006; Stephenson, 2003; Waters & Begley, 2007), want more opportunities to engage in risky activities (Franklin, 2002) and desire more time away from adults supervising their play (Armstrong et al., 2006). What we have argued thus far is that in the last 5 to 10 years, there has been a renewed awakening around children's play specifically focused on outdoor play, a revolt against the standardised playgrounds of the modern era, and a call for encouraging children to get back to nature in our postmodern era (Frost, 2010). Indeed, there are now a growing number of communities, governmental policy directives, NGOs and academic literatures (see Gleave, 2008) devoted to subjects such as balancing risks in children's play, "taking back the streets", encouraging the adoption of independent mobility, free roaming in children (Playing Out, 2017) and getting back to nature (Nature Play, 2017). Initiatives like the *No Child Left Inside Act* in the USA (Frost, 2010) and the *Position Statement* in Canada (ParticipACTION, 2016b) illustrate adults' commitments to the promotion of natural play and learning environments (Frost, 2010) and to encouraging children to play outdoors as much as possible. Gleave (2008) cites a *UK Department of Children, Schools and Families 2008* report stipulating that childhood is a time for learning and exploring, during which children should not to be "wrapped in cotton wool" (p. 24). However, as Opie and Opie (1969) suggested almost 40 years ago, "in the long run, nothing extinguishes self-organised play more effectively than does action to promote it" (p. 10). Today this paradox remains; children's engagement in "free", self-determined play that also involves risk and excitement is stifled (or even "extinguished") through the very public health, education or physical activity interventions that aim to promote it.

These multiple competing and contradictory discourses about risk and play offer what Pronger (2002) calls a salvation narrative. In his critique of the modern technologies of physical fitness, Pronger (2002) argues that salvation is promised through the accumulation of physical activities. With respect to play, children and families are being told they can save themselves (and society) though active and responsible risky outdoor play. In these moments "power is brought to bear on bodies not for the sake of punishing them but for the sake of rescuing, rehabilitating, and saving them" (Rail, 2012, p. 241). We ask this question: is public health's attention on risk, active play and "free-range parenting" promising a salvation on their terms or on children's terms?

As we have demonstrated in this chapter, in contemporary societies – specifically Global North, westernised, industrialised countries – concepts of risk and risk-taking as they are attached to children and their play have come full circle. They have gone from attempts to contain the risks inherent in children's free roaming street play by curbing children's mobility (e.g., through physical education, organised sports, by-laws, built environments etc.) to full on (moral and responsibility) retribution if parents do not encourage their children to engage in risky, physically active outdoor play (ParticipACTION, 2016b). Historically, parents have always been asked by educational, judicial, medical and religious institutions to be dutifully protective in the care of their children (Rose, 1999). Now they are overly critiqued for producing less resourceful children, who are at risk of becoming physically inactive and obese. This critique has been incorporated by new public health agendas around risk and play (e.g., "sedentary play is risky" for your child's health). A set of contradictory discourses has emerged: suggestions that "active play might be risky" and "your child may suffer an injury" are now jettisoned in favour of the belief that risk is necessary. ParticipACTION's *Position Statement* asks this: "If we make injury prevention the ultimate goal of outdoor play space, will there be any fun?" (2016b, p. 1). Thinking about children taking risks in play and particularly playing outdoors requires paying attention to increasingly complex negotiations between parents and children, which are constantly mediated by knowledge of public health discourses and the ever-pervasive media and local discourses about neighbourhood and urban safety, as well as global discourses of health-futurity and citizenship. The *Position Statement* (2016) advocates for a balanced approach where parents, schools, health and injury prevention specialists, governments and the media are asked to consider the long-term dangers and risks of sedentary behaviours above and beyond an "outdated" focus on frivolous injuries, lawsuits, by-laws and sensationalising stories that once elevated cultural fears around children's well-being.

The contradictory discourses about fears and children's play and risk, as noted previously, are historically, politically, socially and culturally contingent. It is important to acknowledge that these discourses and practices have been directed and redirected towards different kinds of play and different kinds of children – a point we will return to in the concluding chapter. Paying close attention to who is responsible for children's risk-taking and health – usually mothers – and who is included and excluded in present calls for children to "freely range" outdoors will be crucial in this contemporary moment when communities are trying to figure out how to protect their children and young people in an era of growing violence, divisiveness and xenophobia, and which is marked by local and global disparities in income distribution (Wells, 2017). If we ignore these systemic and pervasive discourses and practices then *we risk* failing the many children (and parents) at risk of losing free play in the face of government's and public health's biopolitical regimes.

References

Active Health Kids Global Alliance. (2017). *The global matrix 2.0 on physical activity for children and youth*. Retrieved November 2017 from www.activehealthykids.org

Active Healthy Kids Australia Report Card 2016. (2016). *Physical literacy: Do our kids have all the tools?* Retrieved May 2017 from www.activehealthykidsaustralia.com.au/siteassets/documents/ahka-2016-long_form-report-card.pdf

Active Healthy Kids England Report Card 2016. (2016). *Then and now?* Retrieved May 2017 from http://files.site-fusion.co.uk/webfusion119994/file/england_rc_16.pdf

Active Healthy Kids Scotland Report Card 2016. (2016). *Annual review*. Retrieved May 2017 from www.playscotland.org/wp-content/uploads/Play-Scotland-Annual-Review-2016.pdf

Aitken, S. (2001). *Geographies of young people: The morally contested spaces of identity*. London: Routledge.

Alexander, S. A., Frohlich, K. L., & Fusco, C. (2015). 'You have to do 60 minutes of physical activity per day! I saw it on TV': Children's experiences of playing within the context of the public health discourse of playing for health. *Sociology of Health and Illness, 37*(2), 227–240.

Armstrong, S. C., Barker, J., Davey, R., Diosi, M., Horton, J., Kraftl, P., . . . Smith, F. (2006). *Evaluation of play provision and play needs in the London Borough of Redbridge*. London: Redbridge Children's Fund.

Ball, D. (2004). Policy issues and risk-benefit trade-offs of 'safer surfacing' for children's playgrounds. *Accident Analysis and Prevention, 36*, 661–670.

Ball, D. J. (2002). *Playgrounds – risks, benefits and choices. HSE Contract Research Report*, 426/2002. Norwich: HSE Books.

Ball, D., Gill, M., & Spiegal, B. (2008). *Managing risk in play provision: Implementation guide*. London: Play England.

Bartlett, S. (2002). Building better cities with children and youth. *Environment & Urbanization, 14*(2), 3–10.

Beck, U. (1992). *Risk society: Towards a new modernity*. London: Sage Publications.

Benzie, R. (2016, July 11). *Ontario minister urges end to Toronto's road hockey ban*. Retrieved June 2017 from www.thestar.com/news/queensk/2016/07/11/ontario-minister-urges-end-to-torontos-road-hockey-ban.html

Berry, T., Craig, C., Faulkner, G., Latimer, A., Rhodes, R., Spence, J., & Tremblay, M. (2014). Mothers' intentions to support children's physical activity related to attention and implicit agreement with advertisements. *International Journal of Behavioral Medicine*, 21(1), 131–138.

Boero, N. (2009). Fat kids, working moms, and the 'Epidemic of Obesity,: Race, class, and mother blame. In E. Rothblum & S. Solovay (Eds.), *The fat studies reader* (pp. 113–119). New York, NY: New York University Press.

Boesveld, S. (2012, May 4). Return of risk: The growing movement to let kids play like kids. *The National Post*. Retrieved December 2017 from http://nationalpost.com/news/canada/return-of-risk-the-growing-movement-to-let-kids-play-like-kids

Boufous, S., Finch, C., & Bauman, A. (2004). Parental safety concerns: A barrier to sport and physical activity in children? *Australian and New Zealand Journal of Public Health*, 28(5), 482–486.

Boulos, R., Vikre, E., Oppenheimer, S., Chang, H., & Kanarek, R. (2012). ObesiTV: How television is influencing the obesity epidemic. *Physiology & Behavior*, 107(1), 146–153.

Brunelle, S., Coghlan, R., Herrington, S., & Brussoni, M. (2016). Play worth remembering: Are playgrounds too safe? *Child, Youth and Environments*, 26(1), 17–36.

Brussoni, M., Gibbons, R., Gray, C., Ishikawa, T., Sandseter, E. B. H., Bienenstock, A., . . . Tremblay, M. S. (2015). What is the relationship between risky outdoor play and health in children? A systematic review. *International Journal of Environmental Research and Public Health*, 12(6), 6423–6454.

Brussoni, M., Olsen, L., Pike, I., & Sleet, D., (2012). Risky play and children's safety: Balancing priorities for optimal child development. *International Journal of Environmental Research and Public Health*, 9(9), 3134–3148.

Buliung, R., Mitra, R., & Faulkner, G. (2009). Active school transportation in the Greater Toronto Area, Canada: An exploration of trends in space and time (1986–2006). *Preventive Medicine*, 48(6), 507–512.

Burrows, L. (2009). Pedagogizing families through obesity discourse. In J. Wright and V. Harwood (Eds.), *Biopolitics and the obesity "epidemic": Governing bodies* (pp. 127–140). New York, NY: Routledge.

Burrows, L. (2016). Close to home: What kind of family should we become? In S. Dagkas & L. Burrows (Eds.), *Families, young people, physical activity and health: Critical perspectives* (pp. 57–68). London: Routledge.

Canadian Tire. (2013). *We all play for Canada*. Retrieved September 2015 from http://weallplayforcanada.ca/

Carroll-Scott, A. C., Gilstad-Hayden, K., Rosenthal, L., Peters, S., McCaslin, C., Joyce, R., & Ickovicsa, R. J. (2013). Disentangling neighborhood contextual associations with child body mass index, diet, and physical activity: The role of built, socioeconomic, and social environments. *Social Science & Medicine*, 95, 106–114.

Carver, A., Timperio, A., & Crawford, D. (2008). Playing it safe: The influence of neighbourhood safety on children's physical activity – A review. *Health & Place*, 14(2), 217–227.

Carver, A., Veitch, J., Sahlqvist, S., Crawford, D., & Hume, C. (2014). Active transport, independent mobility and territorial range among children residing in disadvantaged areas. *Journal of Transportation Health*, 1(4), 267–273.

Castel, R. (1991). From dangerousness to risk. In G. Burchell, C. Gordon & P. Miller (Eds.), *The Foucault effect: Studies in governmentality* (pp. 281–297). London: Harvester Wheatsheaf.

CBC. (2013, September 17). *Playground equipment involved in rising number of injuries*. Retrieved December 2017 from www.cbc.ca/news/playground-equipment-involved-in-rising-number-of-injuries-1.1858497

CBC. (2016, January 10). *Has old-fashioned fun been trumped by fears of injury and legal action?* Retrieved December 2017 from www.cbc.ca/radio/checkup/has-old-fashioned-fun-been-trumped-by-fears-of-injury-and-legal-action-1.3395495

City News Staff. (2016, June 20). *Trending: Is it time for city hall to overturn the ban on street hockey?* Retrieved July 2017 from http://toronto.citynews.ca/2016/06/20/trending-is-it-time-for-city-hall-to-overturn-the-ban-on-street-hockey/

Cooper, J. (2000). *Listening to children at play*. London: Theories Landscape.

Cosentino, F., & Howell, M. (1971). *A history of physical education in Canada*. Toronto: General Publishing Company Limited.

Coveney, J., & Bunton, R. (2003). In pursuit of the study of pleasure: Implications for health research and practice. *Health: An Interdisciplinary Journal for the Social Study of Health, Illness and Medicine, 7*(2), 161–179.

Crawford, R. (1980). Healthism and the medicalisation of everyday life. *International Journal of Health Services, 19*, 365–388.

Crawford, S., Bennetts, S., Hackworth, N., Green, J., Graesser, H., Cooklin, A., . . . Nicholson, J. M. (2017). Worries, 'weirdos', neighbourhoods and knowing people: A qualitative study with children and parents regarding children's independent mobility. *Health and Place, 45*, 131–139.

Dagkas, S., & Burrows, L. (Eds.). (2016). *Families, young people, physical activity and health: Critical perspectives*. London: Routledge.

Dagkas, S., & Quarmby, T. (2012). Children's embodiment of health and physical capital: The role of the 'pedagogised' family. *Sociology of Sport Journal, 29*, 210–226.

Dean, M. (1999). *Governmentality: Power and rule in modern society*. London: Sage Publications.

Derbyshire, D. (2007). *How children lost the right to roam in four generations*. Retrieved July 2017 from www.dailymail.co.uk/news/article . . . /How-children-lost-right-roam-generations.html

Evans, J., Davies, B., & Wright, J. (2004). *Body knowledge and control: Studies in the sociology of physical education and health*. New York, NY: Routledge.

Faulkner, G., Mitra, R., Buliung, R., Fusco, C., & Stone, M. (2015). Children's outdoor playtime, physical activity, and parental perceptions of the neighbourhood environment. *International Journal of Play, 4*(1), 84–97.

Foucault, M. (1978). *The history of sexuality* (Vol. 1). New York, NY: Random House.

Foucault, M. (1980). *Power/knowledge: Selected interviews and other writings 1972–1977*. New York, NY: Vintage.

Foucault, M. (1991). Governmentality. In G. Burchell, C. Gordon & P. Miller (Eds.), *The Foucault effect: Studies in governmentality* (pp. 87–104). London: Harvester Wheatsheaf.

Fox, N. (1999). *Beyond health: Postmodernism and embodiment*. London: Free Association Books.

Franklin, A. (2002). *Accidents, risk and play in adventure playgrounds in Lambeth, Southwark and Lewisham*. London: National Children's Bureau.

Friedman, M. (2014). Mother blame, fat shame, and moral panic: 'Obesity' and child welfare. *Fat Studies an Interdisciplinary Journal of Body Weight and Society, 4*(1), 14–27.

Frost, J. L. (2005). How playground regulations and standards are messing up children's play. *Today's Playground*, 5(7), 14–19.

Frost, J. L. (2010). *A history of children's play and environments*. New York, NY: Routledge.

Fullagar, S. (2009). Governing healthy family lifestyles. In J. Wright & V. Harwood (Eds.), *Biopolitics and the 'Obesity Epidemic' governing bodies* (pp. 108–126). New York, NY and London: Routledge.

Futures Foundations. (2006). *The changing face of parenting: Professional parenting, information and healthcare*. London: Futures Foundations.

Gainforth, H., Jarvis, J., Berry, T., Chulak-Bozzer, T., Deshpande, S., Faulkner, G., . . . Latimer-Cheung, A. (2015). Evaluating the ParticipACTION 'Think Again' campaign. *Health Education & Behaviour*, 43(4), 434–441.

Gatz, M., Messner, M., & Ball-Rokeach, J. (2002). *Paradoxes of youth and sport*. New York, NY: SUNY.

Gill, T. (2006). Home zones in the UK: History, policy and impact on children and youth. *Children, Youth, Environments*, 16(1), 90–103.

Gill, T. (2007). *No fear: Growing up in a risk society*. London: Calouste Gulbenkian Foundation.

Gill, T. (2009). *Managing risk in play provision: A briefing for risk managers*. London: Play England.

Gill, T. (2010). *Nothing ventured: Balancing risks and benefits in the outdoor*. Nottingham: English Outdoor Council.

Gill, T. (2014). The benefits of children's engagement with nature. A systematic review of literature. *Children, Youth and Environments*, 24(2), 100–134.

Gleave, J. (2008). *Risk and play: A literature review*. London: Play England. Retrieved July 2016 from www.playday.org.uk/PDF/Risk-and-play-a-literature-review.pdf

Go Rving Canada. (2017). *Rediscover you wildhood*. Retrieved July 2017 from https://gorving.ca/bringbackwildhood

Gray, C., Gibbons, R., Larouche, R., Sandseter, E. B. H., Bienenstock, A., Brussoni, M., . . . Tremblay, M. S. (2015). What is the relationship between outdoor time and physical activity, sedentary behaviour, and physical fitness in children? A systematic review. *International Journal of Environmental Research and Public Health*, 12(6), 6455–6474.

Gray, P. (2011). The decline of play and the rise of psychopathology in children and adolescents. *American Journal of Play*, 3(4), 443–463.

Griffin, D. (2015, January 21). Free-range parenting: Easier said than done, but worth the effort. *Huffington Post*. Retrieved August 2017 from www.huffingtonpost.com/daniel-griffin-phd/freerange-parenting-easie_b_6509258.html

Hart, R. (2002). Containing children: Some lessons on planning for play from New York City. *Environment and Urbanization*, 14(2), 135–149.

Heidegger, M. (1954). The question concerning technology. In D.F. Krell (Ed.), *Martin Heidegger: Basic writings* (pp. 283–318). New York: Harper and Row.

Herrington, S., & Nicholls, J. (2007). Outdoor play spaces in Canada: The safety dance of standards as policy. *Critical Social Policy*, 27(1), 128–138. doi:10.1177/0261018307072210

Holloway, S., & Valentine, G. (Eds.). (2000). *Children's geographies: Playing, living, learning*. London: Routledge.

Human Potential Centre. (2015). *State of play survey: Executive report.* Retrieved September 2017 from www.persil.co.nz/wp-content/uploads/sites/10/2015/11/AUT_State_Of_Play-141015.pdf

Ingham, A. (1985). From public issue to private trouble: Well-being and the fiscal crisis of the state. *Sociology of Sport Journal, 2,* 43–55.

International Play Association. (2016). *The child's right to play.* Retrieved July 2017 from http://ipaworld.org/childs-right-to-play/the-childs-right-to-play/

International Play Association. (2017). *Children's right to play and the environment.* Retrieved July 2017 from http://ipaworld.org/childrens-right-to-play-and-the-environment/

Jachyra, P., & Fusco, C. (2016). The place of play: From playground to policy to classroom well-being. *Sport, Education and Society, 21*(2), 217–238. doi:10.1080/13573322.2014.896331

Jackson, D., & Mannix, J. (2004). Giving voice to the burden of blame: A feminist study of mothers' experiences of mother blaming. *International Journal of Nursing Practice, 10*(4), 150–158.

Janssen, I. (2015). Hyper-parenting is negatively associated with physical activity among 7–12 year olds. *Preventative Medicine, 73,* 55–59.

Kirk, D. (1998). *Schooling bodies: School practice and public discourse, 1880–1950.* London: Leicester University Press.

Kirk, D. (2001). Schooling bodies through physical education: Insights from social epistemology and curriculum history. *Studies in Philosophy and Education, 20,* 475–487.

Kremer, S., Trew, K., & Ogle, S. (1997). *Young people's involvement in sport.* London: Routledge.

Ladd-Taylor, M., & Umansky, L. (1998). *"Bad" mothers: The politics of blame in twentieth-century America.* New York, NY: NYU Press.

Landry, S. H. (2005). *Effective early childhood programs: Turning knowledge into action.* Houston, TX: University of Texas at Houston.

LeMoyne, T., & Buchanan, T. (2011). Does 'Hovering' matter? Helicopter parenting and its effect on well-being. *Sociological Spectrum, 31*(4), 399–418.

Lester, S., & Russell, W. (2008). *'Play for a Change'. Play, policy and practice: A review of contemporary perspectives.* London: Play England.

Lester, S., & Russell, W. (2014). Turning the world upside down: Playing as the deliberate creation of uncertainty. *Children, 1,* 241–260.

Lindon, J. (1999). *Too safe for their own good.* London: National Early Years Network.

Louv, R. (2008). *Passage of no child left inside act suggests new era for nature in education.* Retrieved September 2017 from www.childrenandnature.org/2008/09/20/beyond-the-landmark-no-child-left-inside-act/

Lupton, D. (1995). *The imperative of public health: Public health and the regulated body.* London: Sage Publications.

Lupton, D. (1996). *The new public health.* St. Leaonards, Australia: Sage.

Lupton, D. (1999). *Risk.* London: Routledge.

Mangan, J. (1981). *Athleticism in the Victorian and Edwardian public school: The emergence and consolidation of an ideal.* Cambridge: Cambridge University Press.

McIntosh, P. (1968). *Physical education in England since 1800.* London: G. Bell & Sons Ltd.

McNaughton, D. (2011). From the womb to the tomb: Obesity and maternal responsibility. *Critical Public Health*, 21(2), 179–190.

Mehta, D. (2016, July 15). *Game on: Toronto lifts ban on street hockey*. Retrieved July 2017 from www.ctvnews.ca/sports/game-on-toronto-lifts-ban-on-street-hockey-1.2988724

Mitra, R., Faulkner, G., Buliung, R., & Stone, M. (2014). Do parental perceptions of the neighbourhood environment influence children's independent mobility? Evidence from Toronto, Canada. *Urban Studies*, 51(16), 3401–3419.

Moore, R. (1987). Streets as playgrounds. In A. Moudon (Ed.), *Public streets for public use* (pp. 45–62). New York, NY: Van Nostrand Rhinehold.

Morrongiello, B., & Dawber, T. (1998). *Mothers responses to boys and girls engaging in injury risk behaviours on a playground*. Ontario: University of Guelph.

Morrongiello, B., & Lasenby-Lessard, J. (2007). Psychological determinants of risk taking by children: An integrative model and implications for intervention. *Injury Prevention*, 13, 20–25.

Muñoz, S. A. (2009). Children in the outdoors – Literature review. *Sustainable Development Research Centre*. Retrieved July 2016 from www.educationscotland.gov.uk/images/Children in the outdoors literature review_tcm4-597028.pdf

Nature Play. (2017). *Getting our kids outdoors*. Retrieved January 2018 from www.natureplay.org.au

Opie, I., & Opie, P. (1969). *Children's games in the street and playground*. Oxford: Clarendon Press.

Osler, J. (2016, March 30). *Playgrounds begin to focus on riskier play: Some play spaces return to riskier structures to encourage activity*. Retrieved December 2016 from www.cbc.ca/news/canada/playgrounds-risky-play-1.3512559

Parker, G. (2014). Mothers at large: Responsibilizing the pregnant self for the 'Obesity Epidemic'. *An Interdisciplinary Journal of Body Weight and Society*, 3(2), 101–118.

ParticipACTION. (2011). *Think again campaign*. Retrieved June 2012 from www.youtube.com/watch?v=GM7HY2HqXEI&list=PLn9ck0OZhxkYVlk_itMNGnDdS5pqmcTOX&index=6

ParticipACTION. (2015). *The biggest risk is keeping kids indoors: The 2015 ParticipACTION report card on physical activity for children and youth*. Toronto: ParticipACTION.

ParticipACTION. (2016a). *Make room for play*. Retrieved July 15 from www.participaction.com/en-ca/programs/make-room-for-play

ParticipACTION. (2016b). *Position statement on active outdoor play*. Ottawa: ParticipACTION.

ParticipACTION. (2017). *Don't stand between your kids and the great outdoors: Parenting, hovering, risk, outdoors*. Retrieved July 5, 2017 from www.participaction.com/en-ca/blog/kids-parenting/don%27t-stand-between-your-kids-and-the-great-outdoors

Petersen, A., & Lupton, D. (1996). *The new public health: Health and self in the age of risk*. London: Sage Publications.

Petherick, L. (2015). Shaping the child as a healthy child: Health surveillance, schools and biopedagogies. *Cultural Studies – Critical Methodologies*, 15, 361–370.

PlayingOut. (2017). *Make your street a place to play*. Retrieved July 2017 from http://playingout.net

Play Scotland. (2017). *Getting it right for play*. Retrieved September 2017 from www.playscotland.org/wp-content/uploads/assets/Policy-Context.pdf

Pronger, B. (2002). *Body fascism: Salvation in the technology of physical fitness*. Toronto: University of Toronto Press.

Rail, G. (2012). The birth of the obesity clinic: Confessions of the flesh, biopedagogies and physical culture. *Sociology of Sport Journal, 29*(2), 227–253.

Rich, E. (2010a). Editorial: Health surveillance, the body and schooling. *International Journal of Qualitative Studies in Education, 23*, 759–764.

Rich, E. (2010b). Obesity assemblages and surveillance in schools. *International Journal of Qualitative Studies in Education, 23*, 803–821.

Rich, E., & Evans, J. (2009). Performative health in schools: Welfare policy, neoliberalism and social regulation? In J. Wright & V. Harwood (Eds.), *Biopolitics and the obesity epidemic: Governing bodies* (pp. 157–171). Oxon, UK: Routledge.

Riggio, E. (2002). Child friendly cities: Good governance in the best interests of the child. *Environment & Urbanization, 14*(2), 45–58.

Rose, N. (1999). *Governing the soul: The shaping of the private self* (2nd ed.). London: Free Association Books.

Rose, N. (2007). *The politics of life itself: Biomedicine, power, and subjectivity in the Twentieth-First century*. Princeton, NJ: Princeton University Press.

Ryall, E., Russell, W., & MacLean, M. (2013). *The philosophy of play*. London: Routledge.

Sandseter, E. (2009a). Characteristics of risky play. *Journal of Adventure Education and Outdoor Learning, 9*, 3–21.

Sandseter, E. (2009b). Children's expressions of exhilaration and fear in risky play. *Contemporary Issues in Early Childhood, 10*(2), 92–106.

Sandseter, E., & Kennair, L. (2011). Children's risky play from an evolutionary perspective: The anti-phobic effects of thrilling experiences. *Evolutionary Psychology, 9*(2), 257–284.

Scanlan, W. (2017, March 23). *Kids are now heavier, rounder and weaker – The fix ought to be simple*. Retrieved June 2017 from http://ottawasun.com/2017/03/23/scanlan-kids-are-now-heavier-rounder-and-weaker-the-fix-ought-to-be-simple/wcm/78201d1a-486c-4715-a1d2-3bd6db6e1d59

Schoeppe, S., Duncan, M., Badland, H., Oliver, M., & Curtis, C. (2013). Associations of children's independent mobility and active travel with physical activity, sedentary behavior and weight status: A systematic review. *Journal of Science and Medicine in Sport, 16*, 312–319.

Skenazy, L. (2017). *How to raise safe, self-reliant children (without going nuts with worry)*. Retrieved June 2017 from www.freerangekids.com/faq/

Stephenson, A. (2003). Physical risk-taking: Dangerous or endangered? *Early Years, 23*, 35–43.

St. George, D. (2015, June 11). *Maryland officials: Letting 'Free Range' kids walk or play alone is not neglect. Special needs digest*. Retrieved July 2016 from www.specialneedsdigest.com/2015/06/maryland-officials-letting-free-range.html

Stone, M., Faulkner, G., Mitra, R., & Buliung, R. (2014). The freedom to explore: Examining the influence of independent mobility on weekday, weekend and after-school physical activity behaviour in children living in urban and inner-suburban neighbourhoods of varying socioeconomic status. *International Journal of Behavioral Nutrition and Physical Activity, 11*(5).

Taylor, C., Pollard, S., Angus, A., & Rocks, S. (2013). Better by design: Rethinking interventions for better environmental regulation. *Science of the Total Environment*, 447(1), 488–499.

Thompson, C., Travlou, P., & Roe, J. (2006). *Free range teenagers: The role of wild adventure space in young people's lives*. Edinburgh: OPENspace.

Thompson, S. (1999). *Mother's taxi: Sport and women's labour*. New York, NY: SUNY.

Timperio, A., Crawford, D., Telford, A., & Salmon, J. (2004). Perceptions about the local neighborhood and walking and cycling among children. *Preventative Medicine*, 38(1), 39–47.

Tremblay, M. S., Gray, C., Babcock, S., Barnes, J., Bradstreet, C. C., Carr, D., . . . Brussoni, M. (2015). Position statement on active outdoor play. *International Journal of Environmental Research and Public Health*, 12(6), 6475–6505.

Tucker, J. (2017, March 12). *How should our kids play at recess? Alameda schools offer lessons*. Retrieved from www.sfchronicle.com/education/article/How-should-our-kids-play-at-recess-Alameda-10995385.php

Valentine, G. (2004). *Public space and the culture of childhood*. Aldershot: Ashgate.

Valentine, G., & McKendrick, J. (1997). Children's outdoor play: Exploring parental concerns about children's safety and the changing nature of childhood. *Geoforum*, 28(2), 219–235.

Veitch, J., Bagley, S., Ball, K., & Salmon, J. (2006). Where do children usually play? A qualitative study of parents' perceptions of influence on children's active free-play. *Health & Place*, 12(4), 383–393.

Veitch, J., Wang, W.C., Salmon, J., Carver, A., Giles-Corti, B., & Timperio, A. (2017). Who goes to metropolitan parks? A latent class analysis approach to understanding park visitation. *Leisure Sciences*, doi:10.1080/01490400.2017.1325798

Waters, J., & Begley, S. (2007). Supporting the development of risk-taking behaviours in the early years: An exploratory study. *Education*, 35(4), 365–377.

Wells, K. (2017). What does a republican government with Donald Trump as President of the USA mean for children, youth and families? *Children Geographies*, 15(4), 491–497.

Wheway, R. (2008). *Not a risk averse society*. Play Action Online No. 2. March 2008, Fair Play for Children. Retrieved July 2016 from www.fairplayforchildren.org/pdf/1206991484.pdf

Wheway, R., & Millward, A. (1997). *Child's play: Facilitating play on housing estates*. Joseph Rowntree Foundation. Retrieved January 16, 2018 from www.jrf.org.uk/report/childs-play-facilitating-play-housing-estates

Wright, J., & Harwood, V. (Eds.). (2009). *Biopolitics and the obesity epidemic: Governing bodies*. Oxon, UK: Routledge.

Yates, R. (2003). The child friendly cities movement: Its implications for schools and education. *Education Canada*, 43(1), 32, 34–35.

Zamosky, L. (2009). *Free-range parenting: It's a new, hands-off approach to raising kids. Should you give it a try?* Retrieved June 2017 from www.webmd.com/parenting/features/free-range-parenting#1

Zeigler, E. (1979). *History of physical education and sport*. Englewood Cliffs, NJ: Prentice-Hall, Inc.

Chapter 6

Playing just makes me happy

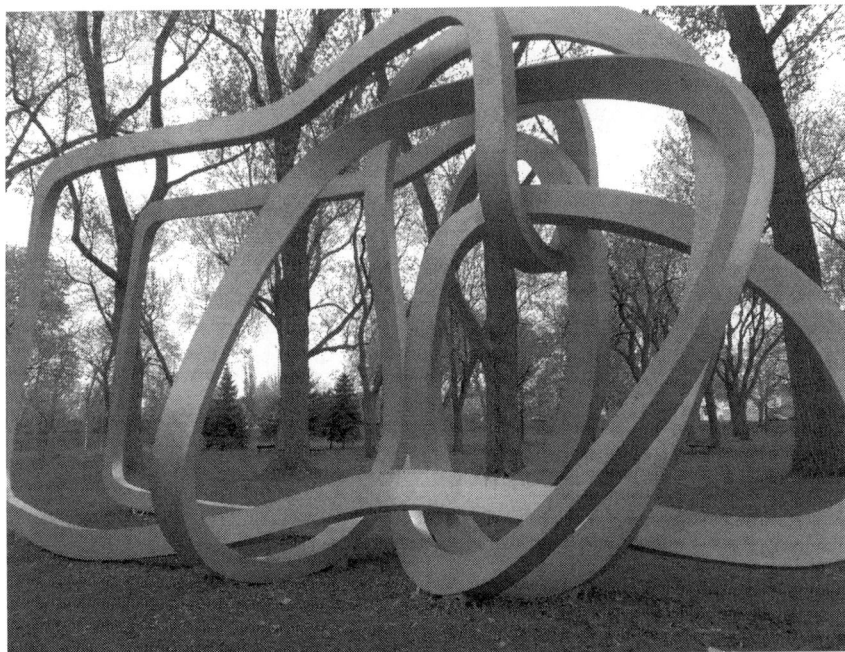

Figure 6.1 Sarah (11 years old) took a photo of a sculpture she likes to climb.

Introduction

Since the conception of this book, ideas about children's play, and the roles of risk and parental involvement in their play, have evolved and changed at lightning pace. It is as though the very interventions into children's play over the last 10 years, some of which are described in this book, have encouraged a re-examination of taken-for-granted assumptions about children's play and led to a questioning of the direction in which children's lives have been changed. In this chapter we return to the idea that playing should simply be fun for children, and in so doing, offer up some definitions and ways of considering play that we think could be helpful in making this goal possible. We will also examine some future developments that may impede this and give some suggestions as to how we, as participants in our respective societies and communities, can strive towards the creation of environments in which children can play in ways that "simply make them happy" (Sutton-Smith, 1997).

Returning to some definitions of play

This book has outlined our exploration of the reasons for why we believe play has been taken up by public health institutions in Canada, and of the ways in which public health's incursion into play might be changing not only how we think about play, but also how play is enacted. We wish to return to some useful definitions of play that have been the mainstay of play descriptions for some time to help remind us of the qualities of play that children often desire.

Feezell's (2013) chapter in Ryall, Russell, and MacLean's (2013) book *The Philosophy of Play* lists a series of useful definitions of play put forward by various play researchers and scholars. The fundamental attributes of these definitions all juxtapose rather abruptly with many of the descriptions of play advanced to reduce childhood obesity and to "get kids moving". For instance, Feezell presents Caillois' (1961) definition of play:

> Play is free (not obligatory); separate (limited in space and time); uncertain (outcomes aren't determined in advance and are due to players' innovations); unproductive (no new goods are created); governed by rules (conventional suspension of ordinary norms); and make-believe (an awareness of the unreality of the play world).
>
> (Caillois, 1961 cited in Feezell, 2013, p. 24)

Feezell also draws on psychologist Stuart Brown's (2009) list of play properties, which he has annotated:

a   Apparently purposeless (done for its own sake)
b   Voluntary ('not obligatory or required by duty')
c   Inherent attraction ("It's fun. It makes you feel good. . . . It's a cure for boredom.")
d   Freedom from time ('When we are fully engaged in play, we lose a sense of the passage of time.')

e   Diminished consciousness of self ("We stop worrying about whether we look good or awkward, smart or stupid. . . . We are fully in the moment, in the zone.")
f   Improvisational potential ("We aren't locked into a rigid way of doing things. We are open to serendipity, to change. . . . The result is that we stumble upon new behaviours, thoughts, strategies, movements, or ways of being.")
g   Continuation desire ("We desire to keep doing it, and the pleasure of the experience drives the desire. We find ways to keep it going. . . . And when it is over, we want to do it again.").

(p. 24)

Ryall et al. (2013) themselves broadly describe play as:

a voluntary activity or occupation executed within certain fixed limits of time and place, according to rules freely accepted but absolutely binding, having its aim in itself and accompanied by a feeling of tension, joy and the consciousness that it is "different" from "ordinary life".

(p. 15)

Despite these definitions, it is perhaps still easier to recognise a true play experience when it is observed or experienced than it is to define it concretely with words. For instance, it is through having played freely oneself or by having observed others at "free" play that we can understand that play indeed has its aim "in itself", involves "tension, joy" and is "different" from "ordinary life". Importantly, we can recognise that these definitions and descriptions of play experiences are significantly different from the forms of play that are prescribed for health, or that have a particular instrumental value. Indeed, they underscore the strong contrast between play as ideally defined and the kind of productive play being promoted to children within public health.

We have examined, though the lens of play, physical activity and public health, how children have become the target of social, political, educational and legal regulations that constitute children as the powerless and dependent other in relation to adults in society (Lester & Russell, 2014). Their every movement must be regulated; even their moments of play, which have traditionally been largely unmonitored, now require increased surveillance. We find that this increased regulation of childhood is accompanied by a movement away from the question of *what* children play to the instrumental investigation of *where* and *why* they play. This shift in focus demonstrates that rather than being concerned with *what* children want to be playing, many adults have become more concerned with *where* we want children to be and *how* and *what* we want children to become through their play. As described in Chapter 3, it was Brian Sutton-Smith (1997) who famously termed this "play as progress". Sutton-Smith writes: "play effectively becomes privileged over work both as a learning or arousal-seeking activity and as a major factor in the individual's mental and emotional development" (p. 141).

As we have discussed in our book, societal trends and adult biases and fears have increasingly regulated and controlled play, suppressing activities deemed inappropriate, aggressive or dangerous, and encouraging activities considered productive, beneficial or therapeutic. This attempt to govern play implies that play is something that can be subordinated to both adult and children's own intentions. Throughout our book we added to pre-existing critiques of the instrumentalisation of play by exploring what we call the public healthification of play, a new twist on the control of play by making it useful for physical health purposes (and obesity reduction, in particular).

We argue that when play is left alone – engaged in without an explicit purpose – it may nonetheless be of benefit to children's well-being, whether this be social, emotional, psychological or even physical well-being. Indeed, until recently, children's play was one of the last social activities where uncertainty was permitted (Caillois, 1961; Lester & Russell, 2014). The reason we are concerned with the paradox we raise in this book with regard to public health incursions into play is that in the long run, as Russell (2013) suggests, "nothing extinguishes self-organised play more effectively than does action to promote it" (p. 166).

New definitions of play: risky play, real play and active outdoor play

In preparing the materials for this book it became increasingly apparent to us that the views on how to intervene on children's health and physical well-being through play were changing faster than we could write. Over the course of several years, what began as a rhetoric involving fears for children's safety in outdoor play and very prescribed ways of being physically active, such as those suggested by *Active Healthy Kids Canada* and the *Active Healthy Kids Global Alliance* (2014), had transitioned. Suddenly there was a new concern; parents were being told to allow their children to take educated risks and that they themselves were to "turn a blind eye" on what their children were doing when playing. As we discussed in Chapter 5, we found that there were suddenly new definitions of play that were more inclusive of what has been termed risky play; a form of play designed, in part, to counter parents' constant gaze (e.g., helicopter parenting).

Ellen Sandseter (2009), a trend-setter for this idea of risky play, has identified what she considers its six main components: 1) play at great heights; 2) play with high speed; 3) play with dangerous tools; 4) play near dangerous elements; 5) rough-and-tumble play; and 6) play where children can disappear. These new definitions of "risky" play, while seeking to be less restrictive for children, still seemingly suggest a health purpose and in some ways also represent new prescriptions for how to play. Moreover, along with these definitions has come a push to operationalise and measure active play. Paradoxically, even a critical perspective on the incursion into children's play is an "involvement" and an active attempt to shape a particular kind of children's play.

One of the most illustrative examples of this new trend regarding children's play is found in a 2015 report prepared by the *Human Potential Centre* (2015) at the Auckland University of Technology in New Zealand entitled *State of Play Survey: Executive Report*. In this report the authors adopt the term "real play" to designate what they call a shift in perspective concerning play. The authors write that a return to a "real play" culture allows children the freedom to play creatively on their own terms, balancing exposure to risk with potential developmental benefits. Real play is described as any play that involves risky play à la Sandseter (play involving rough-and-tumble activities, speed, heights, natural elements, tools or independent exploration) and object play (play that uses loose parts or objects to construct, move or interact with others). This type of "real play" integrates the fears voiced by parents over the last 10–15 years that play of this sort could be dangerous with new attempts to shift the discourse to encourage parents (and society more broadly) to allow children to engage in the same risks that were once feared and avoided.

The justification for allowing the reintegration of risks into children's play, however, is not just to make play more fun, free and unstructured. Indeed, this report makes clear that "real play" is associated with a range of positive physical and mental health outcomes, including increases in physical activity, social skills, resilience, creativity, risk management skills and a decrease in anxiety. The report even suggests that "real play" has been linked to increased executive functions in children, an advanced cognitive system essential for planning, problem-solving, inhibitory control and managing novel or potentially dangerous situations. Lastly, and perhaps most importantly for our risk-adverse society, the authors of this report suggest that providing "real play" opportunities for children does not increase the prevalence of injuries.

Similarly, in Canada a diverse cross-sectorial group of researchers and partners representing 14 organisations, as well as more than 1,600 stakeholders, collaborated to develop and revise the evidence-informed *Position Statement on Active Outdoor Play* for children aged 3–12 (Position Statement on Active Outdoor Play, 2016). The *Position Statement*, which we began describing in Chapter 5, was in part a response to the polarising debate between opposing positions on play. On the one hand, *Active Healthy Kids Canada* and its supporters wanted to ensure that children were given the opportunity to be as fully physically active as often as possible. Part of their campaign to achieve this was found in their 2012 *Active Healthy Kids Canada Report Card* in which they supported self-directed, active outdoor play for children (Active Healthy Kids Canada, 2012). On the other hand, a contemporaneous *Canadian Paediatric Position Statement* (Fuselli & Yanchar, 2012) focused on preventing playground injuries by emphasising the importance of the active supervision of children and was accompanied by practitioner, academic, legal and insurance-led concerns regarding the potential harms of active (including risky) outdoor play.

The *Position Statement on Active Outdoor Play* begins with a provocative introduction designed to clearly suggest an either/or situation:

> In an era of schoolyard ball bans and debates about safe tobogganing, have we as a society lost the appropriate balance between keeping children healthy and active and protecting them from serious harm? If we make too many rules about what they can and can't do, will we hinder their natural ability to develop and learn? If we make injury prevention the ultimate goal of outdoor play spaces, will there be any fun? Are children safer sitting on the couch instead of playing actively outside? We need to recognize the difference between danger and risk. And we need to value long-term health and fun as much as we value safety.
> (Position Statement, 2016, p. 1)

The authors bring forth evidence in the *Position Statement* that 1) when children are outside they move more, sit less and play longer; 2) outdoor play is safer than society currently thinks; 3) there are nefarious health consequences to keeping kids indoors; 4) hyper-parenting limits physical activity and can harm mental health; 5) when children are closely supervised outside, they are less active and, finally, 6) outdoor play that occurs in minimally structured, free and accessible environments facilitates socialisation with peers, the community and the environment, reduces feelings of isolation, builds inter-personal skills and facilitates healthy development (pp. 1–2). The recommendations concluding the *Position Statement* range from encouraging parents to permit their children to engage more fully with their outdoor environments in a variety of weather conditions, to stimulating Canadian Provincial and Municipal governments to work together to create an environment where public entities are protected from frivolous lawsuits over minor injuries related to normal and healthy outdoor risky active play.

Given these fascinating and rapid developments in the conception of what "appropriate" play should be for children and how it is defined, we wondered whether the problem we posed at the beginning of the book had been resolved; researchers, schools, organisations and governments are understanding that kids just need to be left alone to play in the ways they desire. The rest of the chapter explores some future anticipated concerns we have with this new openness to play as well as some unresolved issues.

Measuring active play

Among the various and potentially problematic outcomes of children's play continuing to be under the gaze of public health research are the new attempts to measure it. Now that there seems to be an increasingly established relationship between "active play" and physical activity levels, there is a desire to develop the best indicator for "active play" in order to further substantiate its beneficial effects on physical health. In a recently published Canadian systematic review of active play measures (Truelove, Vanderloo, & Tucker, 2017), the authors suggest that active play and physical activity are frequently used synonymously. The review comes out of a concern that a clearly defined, operationalised and measurable term would make active play easier to encourage, rather than focusing on physical activity promotion alone.

And this is key for these authors. Given the relative failures within Canada of promoting physical activity at a population level, and with the growing obesity rates and reductions in play, researchers are desperate to help Canadian children become more physically active. The promotion of active play, as we have discussed throughout this book, seems to be a promising avenue. Indeed, the promotion of active play has been reported to increase physical activity, and as mentioned in Chapter 3, active play was headlined in the Canadian 2012 *ParticipACTION Report Card on Physical Activity*. But what is particularly striking about Truelove et al.'s (2017) systematic review is the emphasis they place on the importance of framing physical activity differently (through the term active play) in order to make it palatable. The authors of the review claim that from a public health perspective, active play may be easier to promote to young children than strictly activities defined as physical activity. This, they argue, may be the case because there is less emphasis on intensity with active play and more on having fun while moving around, without necessarily requiring structured programming or specific equipment. They suggest that the importance of advocating for active play is relevant for childcare staff as well, particularly as staff have previously identified the challenges of facilitating physical activity in childcare settings. Truelove et al. (2017) suggest that the encouragement of active play may be more feasible and less daunting and, therefore, prove helpful in supporting the increased accumulation of physical activity in settings outside of the home. The review authors suggest that active play is defined in most of the literature as a form of physical activity, and, indeed, only two studies included in the review described active play as involving fun behaviour. Definitions included terms such as these:

> gross motor movement, unstructured activity, freely chosen, and occurs outside. Examples of active play behaviours included: swinging, climbing, pulling, balancing, jumping, rolling, running and skipping.
>
> (p. 162)

The authors of the review suggest a working definition to help with the operationalisation of active play. They define it as "a form of gross-motor or total body movement in which young children exert energy in a freely chosen, fun, and unstructured manner". They then further recommend that:

> a tool (i.e., questionnaire) be designed which captures the type of activity (e.g., running, playing, etc.), the location of the play (e.g., indoor, outdoor, etc.) as well as the motivation behind young children's active play behaviour, as it is meant to be a fun, unstructured and freely chosen form of physical activity.
>
> (p. 164)

Coupling this tool with an objective measure of activity (i.e., accelerometry) which accesses the duration and intensity of active play is thus seen to be essential to researchers, childcare providers and parents in order to help encourage young children to participate in active play daily.

However, having another take on the growing popularity of the concept of "active play" for children, Lester and Russell (2014) have suggested that the identification, measurement and classification of activities, such as active play, is a driving force of neo-liberalism. Ryall et al. (2013) suggest that the dominant developmentalist paradigm for understanding childhood as a preparation for adulthood, as we have discussed in our book, has fed the growth of standardised and technical interventions into the lives of children, such as attempting to measure their play. This, it is suggested, may be to the detriment of a more holistic approach regarding children's play. Studies such as those conducted by MacDougall, Schiller, and Darbyshire (2004) and Darbyshire, MacDougall, and Schiller (2005) in Australia, as well as our own study, show that when children are asked about the meaning of play, they immediately distinguish it from sport, physical activity and fitness. For the participants in MacDougall et al.'s (2004) study, descriptors used by children, and associated with play, included "fun", "spontaneity", "interactions with friends", "not too competitive" and "not too aggressive". Those associated with physical activity, on the other hand, included "running around", "muscle building", "weight lifting" and various sports. Responses to the idea of play also elicited a sense of neighbourhood and community not present when children described physical activity or sport.

In our own study, children offered the similar descriptors of what they liked about playing. Some suggested playing is when "you do whatever you want", when "it's me who chooses what I do" and when "there are no limits". Other children used expressions to describe what they liked about playing specifically: "not necessarily funny, but it's something that interests me", or to describe the affective effect a particular activity had on them: "when I'm angry or I'm sad, I draw and it calms me down", or it gives "some time to rest". These descriptors of play activities as including choice, fewer limits, interest, calm or rest differ from, and are more varied than, those most often described by public health experts promoting the benefits of active play. Indeed, the descriptions of play provided by children in our study did not always involve "active play" or forms of play that fulfilled criteria for physical activity. Furthermore, such descriptions defy measurement and quantification, potentially leaving active play promoters, and those attempting to measure play, in a bit of a conundrum.

Commodification of play

We wish to turn briefly here to the issue of commodification in the discussion on play as we feel it plays a crucial role that must continue to be scrutinised if we are we to move away from some of the more confined or limiting notions of play to which we have become accustomed today. Indeed, we view an important part of what has happened to play over the past few decades to be due to its commodification and commercialisation. In earlier chapters, we have briefly touched on the phenomenon of baby gyms, electronic or screen-play, and other ways in which children's play has been commercialised, that is, made into a product legitimised through one's ability to pay for it.

For instance, Freund and Martin's (2004) evaluation of the contemporary drive towards "fitness" in adults (i.e., "defined in the sense of 'being able to' . . . the psychosocial capacity to engage in various activities, working, moving" p. 264) has an interesting analogy to the discourse on play. In their article they suggest that "fitness" is not integrated into people's everyday lives, but slotted in as a "task", one that is privatised and commodified (i.e., paid for in private spaces). Similar to the description of the role of consumption and fitness for adults, Evans and Davies (2010) describe the turn towards the commercialisation of play for children as a means of social improvement. They describe how, in contemporary culture, there is increasing concern with the "work of learning" in order for children to become appropriately physically literate in physical activity and sport. Parents are enrolling their children in such activities as PEPE (private enterprise physical education) to ensure that their children develop complex sets of physical, social and intellectual skills through programmes of structured informality (play), which are meant to prepare them socially and physically for life. What's more, these courses are not just geared towards children's betterment, but "play" on parental concerns that *not* taking part in such activities is an abrogation of their parental responsibility – a form of neglect. The continued commodification of children's play, even if in some situations it is ostensibly to improve children's physical health and "fitness" (i.e., through active gaming, for instance), has to be continually questioned for what else these activities advance (i.e., financial gains), how it transforms children's leisure (i.e., "fun" as something that can be purchased) and at what cost (i.e., what other non-tangible elements of play and pleasure it may negate).

In a similar way, Neil Postman argued in the 1980s in his book *The Disappearance of Childhood* that communication technologies generally, and television in particular, are having significant (and negative) effects on children and ideas we have about "childhood". Television, he argued, with undistinguished programming targeting adults and children in similar ways, has erased the line between what we consider to be an adult and a child, as well as what we accept and treat as adult and child behaviour (Postman, 1994). This meant that children, in terms of language, dress, activities and general leisure pursuits, were in many ways no different from, and were not treated differently than, adults. Viewing changes to childhood in this light, it would perhaps not be surprising then, in terms of children's leisure and physical activities, to see "Little Gyms" for children or children's fitness centres emerging alongside – and in some ways indistinguishable from – those created for adults.

We critically note the commercialisation of play here for how it may negatively affect children's engagement with play activities, and there is no doubt that television and its popularity as a tool of entertainment has had a role in the reframing of children's play activities. However, we also understand the notions of childhood and children's play as being in constant flux, as part of historically and socially situated contingencies, and therefore not as an ideal and desired state that we believe children's play ought to return to. As we come to in the next section, we discuss the caution we take in referring to nostalgic ideas of childhood and play of the past.

Problems of harking back to the past (nostalgia)

While throughout this book we have clearly been supporting the idea that children should be free to play on their own terms, we are also cautious of calls for a "return" to the lifestyles and characteristics of the past. Researchers have extolled the virtues of lifestyles of the past because, in relation to mainstream western societies, children and adults alike were comparatively active and thus resistant to obesity (Tremblay et al., 2005, 2008; Postman, 1994). There are multiple problems with harkening back to a specific tradition or to the past, however, as it ignores many of the social and cultural exclusions with respect to who was able to play and where they were able to play.

Moreover, the kind of nostalgia that valorises "getting back to nature" also assumes that nature is in and of itself an untouched and idealised space, instead of a place for public consumption. As Hermer (2002) argues "nature has been organized as a political object in modern life" (p. 119). Indeed, if we are to embrace the idea(l)s of children exploring their "wildhoods" (GORving, 2017), it is important to ask, who it is that has the right to wander (Donnelly, 1993)?

> *Nature* has been defined for us in particular ways, and we have been prevented from access in order to conserve that definition of nature. Ideas of *privacy* and *private property* have been constructed in order

to preserve those "rights" for the privileged, and to deny access to land because of the potential violation of privacy and in order to affirm the "private" nature of property. Finally, *land use* has also been defined in order to exclude.

(Donnelly, 1993, p. 190, emphasis in original)

While this may seem to step outside our focus on play and public health, we believe that it is worth noting. There are political, cultural, social and spatial histories to public health presumptions about play, and it is incumbent on critical play researchers to unpack these assumptions. We want to acknowledge that when heritage and nostalgia are emphasised, they can re-inscribe geographies and histories of empire and settler-colonialism which reproduce and naturalise relations of domination. In Canada (and we recognise that this has happened in many other places such as USA, Australia, Africa etc.) any harkening back to the past and "nature" ignores violent settler-colonialism and the eradication of Indigenous and Aboriginal cultures that has occurred over the last 150–200 years (Hudson-Rodd, 1998; Razack, 2002). Historically, children and young people who could play outside and could roam freely – Indigenous children and youth – have ended up being the most confined through settler-colonial practices (i.e., reserves, residential schools), all of which has destroyed their own histories of play and physical activity (Norman et al., 2015).

Additionally, as we have alluded to elsewhere in this book, the containment of children's play historically has been directed at poor and racialised children and youth, and these are children and youth who have been depicted as dangerous and polluting of the body politic (Goldberg, 1993). Yet, paradoxically, many poor and racialised children and youth may have had more access to free play and outdoors because their families were not able to afford the equipment needed for sports participation or were unable to access sports because of the legacies of blatant racism in youth sports (Fleming, 2016; Sheerder & Vandermeerschen, 2016). However, most often these children and youth live in environments that do not support such free roaming play (Canada Parks and Recreation Association, 2005; Fusco, 2007, 2012; MacDonald, Abbott, Knez, & Nelson, 2009) or they are subjected to harassment from authorities (Wortley & Owusu-Bempah, 2014) or they are surrounded by dilapidated infrastructure that make it impossible to play and wander freely (Silk & Andrews, 2006). The *Position Statement on Active Outdoor Play* (2016) in Canada does state that it "applies to girls and boys (aged 3–12) regardless of ethnicity, race, or family socioeconomic status" and that "children who have a disability or medical condition should also enjoy active outdoor play in compliance with guidance from a health professional" (p. 1). However, this statement fails to take into account the intersectionality[1] of children and youth's lives and how the conditions and spaces of some of these children's lives (i.e., street violence, lack of play spaces, children caretaking other children (usually girls), lack of family resources, recently immigrated) may prevent them from engaging in play in their neighbourhoods (Fine & Ruglis, 2009; Fitzpatrick & LaGory, 2003; Sabo & Veliz, 2008; Taylor & Doherty, 2005; Wexler & Eglinton, 2015). Given these circumstances, it may be middle-class children and youth who are most likely to benefit from the calls to get outside and into nature, although there is some reason to believe that recent "helicopter parenting" trends are classed and that middle and upper-middle class children may indeed be those least likely to have freedom in their play. We can, however, only speculate that all the qualities that are associated with outdoor play – resilience, autonomy, confidence, problem-solving – may be presumed to reside in certain children more than others (Azzarito & Macdonald, 2016).

We believe it is important to think about whom this new public healthification of play is directed towards. While there have always been incursions into the lives of children under the guise of protection and reform (Cavallo, 1981; Frost, 2010; Baker, 2001), it is important to ask some of the following questions, adapted from Lupton (1999): what kinds of subjects are now being constructed through discourses on play? How are new discourses on play emerging and supplanting other discourses, and what are the effects of this for knowledges and subjects of play? (p. 33). While we certainly support the idea(l) of children taking risks and playing outside as they are taking back the streets, critical questions still need to be addressed: what is the idealised play outdoors composed of? What is desired in this play? And, who is imagined to participate in this play?

Furthermore, while the trend to get children playing outside and moving is clearly well-intentioned, we believe, to paraphrase Wall (2013), that it aligns with popular discourses and practices of social discipline and individualism. These approaches to play may also be problematic because they "discourage experimenting with desires and imagination in ways that might open up new meanings and relations" (Wall, 2013, p. 35). Referring to notions similar to the nostalgic in play, Wall (2013) argues that when play and childhood are over-sentimentalised, "children's actual lives are stripped of human struggle and complexity" and "the complexity of children's play experiences" are obscured (p. 36). Moreover, an epidemiological view of risky outdoor play, which is cultivated by some of the physical activity *Report Cards* and the *Position Statements*, appears to take a rather "scientific approach to the Other [the child]" who is "treated as an object to be observed and examined from a distance for the purpose of anticipating some future behaviour [a life of physical fitness through play]" (Vilhauer, 2013, p. 80). Lester (2013) suggests that the danger of steering minds and bodies towards "a knowable destiny" stifles creative possibilities and the remarkability and novelty of play (p. 134).

The globalisation of play: perspectives from the global north

With the expansion of *Active Healthy Kids Canada Report Cards* into a *Global Alliance* (2014) there is an urgency to examine how contemporary western perspectives on play, physical activity and movement may be re-inscribing power relationships.

As briefly touched on in the book already, a *Global Alliance* was developed by Canadian researchers in 2014 to expand the *Report Cards for Physical Activity* to countries around the world. By 2016 there were already 38 countries participating in the *Global Alliance* all of whom had created their own version of the *Report Card* (see www.activehealthykids.org/registered-countries/). The impetus behind the expansion of the *Report Cards* came from various sources, among others, from research conducted by the *World Health Organisation* (WHO, 2010, 2016). The WHO (2010) suggested that alongside childhood obesity concerns in countries of the global north, middle- and lower-income countries of the global south were also beginning to experience significant increases in childhood obesity, and that this looming epidemic had to be actively addressed. They developed a set of *Global Recommendations on Physical Activity for Health* (2010), which included a section specifically recommending appropriate levels of physical activity for children and youth, globally.

With regard to the countries of the global south specifically, the WHO (2016) later argued that an additional obstacle to reducing obesity among children in these countries was the socio-cultural differences regarding what it means to be a "healthy child". They write:

> Childhood obesity is often under-recognized as a public health issue in these settings, where, culturally, an overweight child is often considered to be healthy.
>
> (WHO, 2016, p. 2)

As such, in creating the *Global Alliance*, the aim of this work, according to the director of the *Alliance*, Mark Tremblay, was to exchange ideas and methods for combatting childhood obesity between participating countries. The goal of the *Global Alliance* was to:

> expand our work as a global community of childhood PA researchers and advocates to learn from one another and challenge conventional within country solutions with international cross-fertilization of ideas and approaches.
>
> (Tremblay et al., 2014, p. S122)

Concretely, becoming a member of the *Global Alliance* meant that each country had to fulfil a set of conditions that would help to streamline the measurement, evaluation and comparison of children's physical activity across countries. This implied following the same standardised methodology to find data on children's physical activity, to evaluate at least the nine principal indicators using the best available country data, and to write and publish a *Report Card for Physical Activity* for one's respective country.

With the results published in each country's *Report Card*, the *Global Alliance* produced a *Global Matrix* of graded physical activity indicators, which can then be analysed and compared across countries. According to Tremblay et al. (2014), the *Global Matrix* of grades:

> assesses global variation in indicators related to PA, but also serves as a tool to motivate change, facilitate advocacy, and cross-fertilize efforts aimed at empowering *the movement to get kids movin-garound the world.
>
> (pp. S113–S114)

While the intention of the *Global Alliance* is again to respond to the calls made by the WHO and other global physical activity organisations (e.g., *Global Observatory for Physical Activity*) and help to combat the growth of childhood obesity worldwide, there are a few concerns we wish to highlight. For example, these "solutions" to obesity, developed in the global north and introduced globally, may create new problems in countries where these problems were not formerly present. That is, through the introduction of *Report Cards*, including the methodology, the measurement, the concepts and the underlying values around health and childhood, new problems regarding children's physical health and their leisure activities may be produced.

Merry (2016) writes about the creation of problems through the creation and measurement of indicators in her book *The Seductions of Quantification* (2016). She argues that the process alone of measuring something tends to produce the phenomenon it claims to measure (Merry, 2016 p. 12). In the case of the *Report Cards for Physical Activity*, it is therefore possible that measuring and evaluating a concept such as "active play" for obesity prevention (a main indicator in the *Report Card*) in a country where neither the concept nor the problem of obesity exist, may indeed create new phenomena and new problems around children's physical heath and their leisure lives. Moreover, and not to be neglected, the urgent promotion of physical activity and "active play" may, in some countries, come at the expense of attending to other pressing concerns, such as poverty, malnutrition and the destruction of public spaces in which to play.

Conclusion: initiatives incorporating this critique

Children have been called an indicator species for cities. The visible presence of children and youth of different ages and backgrounds, with and without their parents, outside in city streets, sidewalks, yards and open spaces is a sign of the health of human habitats. Indeed, the extent to which neighbourhoods, cities and towns support children's outdoor play – i.e., its "playability" – can be directly linked not only to children's health, levels of obesity and psychological well-being, but also to the population's well-being as a whole. We end this book on an optimistic note as numerous recent initiatives on children's play and city life lead us to believe that there are attempts to concretely learn from past trends that confined or regulated play, and that are beginning to understand the importance of creating spaces within which children can play without necessarily prescribing what, how, when or with whom to play.

For instance, healthy city experiments, such as the Woonerfs in the Netherlands, or Home Zones in the UK, provide a space for cars while fully accommodating the social and physical needs of residents (i.e., children and adults) through the physical alteration and redesign of city streets. These initiatives improve the quality of life in residential areas by designing them with people in mind, not just for traffic; the street is shared among pedestrians, children, cyclists and motor vehicles; however, people have the ultimate priority over vehicular traffic. Recent initiatives in Canada are also an encouraging sign that concern about children's play is becoming more of a conduit for change in cityscapes than is the placement of responsibility for play on parents or than prescriptions for families for how to parent properly. The *Public Health Agency of Canada* has recently released a report entitled, *Designing Healthy Living* (2017), in which a call for multi-sectoral approaches has been made to help develop the links between neighbourhood designs and physical and mental health and overall well-being.

Furthermore, the Lawson Foundation's *Outdoor Play Strategy* (2016), a $2.8 million strategy, has funded multiple partners across Canada and created a multi-sectoral effort to address children's outdoor play opportunities nationally. As part of their strategy, 14 initiatives focusing on "play strategies" were funded to concretely improve children's play possibilities in local spaces. These initiatives aim to produce tools and training that will inform policies, practitioners and decision makers as a way to support children's outdoor play on topics ranging from "physical activity, recreation, injury prevention, public health, early childhood education, environment, education, mental health, but all focused on children's outdoor play" (Outdoor Play Strategy, Lawson Foundation, 2016).

Other research in England and Wales, for instance, has been conducted by Russell, Lester, Smith, MacLean and Williams on the memories of adventure playgrounds that children, families and communities had, to explore the value of these playgrounds. The project entitled *Sharing Memories of Adventure Play* (SMAP, 2016) draws on various innovative methodologies (i.e., post-qualitative research methodologies such as memory studies, geography, philosophy and policy) to develop a new methodology called "critical cartography" to valorise different characteristics of adventure playgrounds in order to inform future policies around play. Critical to their research is that rather than emphasise the instrumental value of adventure playgrounds (ability to address concerns around physical inactivity, obesity, crime), the diverse stories they gathered brought to the fore other kinds of value that adventure playgrounds have for children and adults (e.g., linked to moods, habits, rituals and feelings of safety, of being oneself, care and acceptance), characteristics that are otherwise obscured by more instrumental notions of adventure playgrounds.

We conclude our book mentioning these ongoing projects, and some of our own subsequent work on play (research addressing children and their parents, SSHRC, 2011–2014), as well as recent international research collaborations examining urban landscapes and the creation of "playable" spaces in cities because all of these projects provide an optic of children's play that is less filled with concern about its decline, than with the prospect of opening up new possibilities for play. Indeed, while some of these initiatives continue to focus on the promotion of outdoor play, they also imply new approaches, new methodologies and incorporate past critiques, and, in doing so, they not only directly affect the local spaces for children's outdoor leisure possibilities, but they also help to redirect discussions of play towards the creation of leisure that is less goal-directed, less instrumental and that includes new possibilities for children, families and the broader population to engage in play. As discussions around children's play gain further momentum, and as they incorporate past critiques, the discourses and possibilities for "thinking" about leisure, play, fun and childhood also expand and change. It is with these future discussions, possibilities and debates that we hope to continue to engage.

Note

1 Intersectionality as a concept enables researchers to recognise that we are simultaneously members of many groups, and people's complex identities can shape the specific way they experience discrimination. It also refers to the fact that forms of oppression, like racism, classism, sexism and xenophobia are actually mutually dependent and intersecting in nature, and together they compose a unified system of oppression (Crenshaw, 1995).

References

Active Healthy Kids Canada. (2012). *Is active play extinct? Report card on physical activity for children and youth*. Toronto, Canada: Active Healthy Kids Canada.

Active Healthy Kids Global Alliance. (2014). *Global alliance*. Retrieved March 2017 from www.activehealthykids.org/about-us

Azzarito, L., & Macdonald, D. (2016). Unpacking gender/sexuality/race/disability/social class to understand the embodied experiences of young people in physical culture. In K. Green & A. Smith (Eds.), *Routledge handbook of youth sport* (pp. 321–331). Oxon, UK: Routledge.

Baker, B. M. (2001). *In perpetual motion: Theories of power, educational history and the child*. New York, NY: Peter Lang Publishing.

Brown, S. (2009). *Play: How it shapes the brain, opens the imagination, and invigorates the soul*. Toronto: Penguin Group.

Caillois, R. (1961). *Man, play, games* (M. Barash, Trans.). Urbana, IL: University of Illinois Press.

Canada Parks and Recreation Association. (2005). *National policy: Access to recreation for low-income families*. Retrieved September 2015 from https://lin.ca/sites/default/files/attachments/EverybodyGetstoPlayPositionPaper.pdf

Cavallo, D. (1981). *Muscles and morals: Organized playgrounds and urban reform 1880–1920*. Philadelphia, PA: University of Pennsylvania Press.

Crenshaw, K. W. (1995). Mapping the margins: Intersectionality, identity politics, and violence against women of color. In K. Crenshaw, N. Gotanda, G. Peller & K. Thomas

(Eds.), *Critical race theory: The key writings that formed the movement* (pp. 357–383). New York, NY: New Press.

Darbyshire, P., MacDougall, C., & Schiller, W. (2005). Multiple methods in qualitative research with children: More insight or just more? *Qualitative Research, 5*(4), 417–436.

Donnelly, P. (1993). The right to wander: Issues in the leisure use of countryside and wilderness areas. *International Review for the Sociology of Sport, 28*(2–3), 187–201.

Engle Merry, S. (2016). *The seductions of quantification: Measuring human rights, gender violence, and sex trafficking.* Chicago, IL: The University of Chicago Press.

Evans, J., & Davies, B. (2010). Family, class and embodiment: Why school physical education makes so little difference to post-school participation patterns in physical activity. *International Journal of Qualitative Studies in Education, 23*(7), 765–784.

Feezell, R. (2013). A pluralist conception of play. In E. Ryall, W. Russell & M. MacLean (Eds.), *The philosophy of play* (pp. 11–31). London: Routledge.

Fine, M., & Ruglis, J. (2009). Circuits and consequences of dispossession: The racialized realignment of the public sphere for U.S. youth. *Transforming Anthropology, 17*(1), 20–33.

Fitzpatrick, K., & LaGory, M. (2003). Placing health in urban sociology: Cities as mosaics of risk and protection. *City and Community, 2*(1), 33–46.

Fleming, S. (2016). Youth sport, race and ethnicity. In K. Green & A. Smith (Eds.), *Routledge handbook of youth sport* (pp. 287–296). Oxon, UK: Routledge.

Freund, P., & Martin, G. (2004). Walking and monitoring: Fitness and the social organisation of movement. *Sociology of Health and Illness, 26*(3), 273–286.

Frost, J. L. (2010). *A history of children's play and play environments: Toward a contemporary child-saving movement.* New York, NY: Routledge.

Fusco, C. (2007). 'Healthification' and the promises of urban space: A textual analysis of representations of place, activity, youth (PLAY-ing) in the city. *International Review for the Sociology of Sport, 423*(1), 43–63.

Fusco, C. (2012). Governing PLAY: Moral geographies, healthification and neoliberal urban imaginaries. In D. Andrews & M. Silk (Eds.), *Sport and neo-liberalism* (pp. 143–159). Philadelphia, PA: Temple University Press.

Fuselli, P., & Yanchar, N. L. (2012). Preventing playground injuries. *Paediatrics & Child Health, 17*, 328–330.

Goldberg, D. (1993). Polluting the body politic: Race and urban location. In *Racist culture* (pp. 185–205). Malden, MA: Blackwell Publishing Inc.

GoRving Canada. (2017). *Rediscover your wildhood.* Retrieved July 2017 from https://gorving.ca/bringbackwildhood/

Hermer, J. (2002). *Regulating Eden.* Toronto, ON, Canada: University of Toronto Press.

Hudson-Rodd, N. (1998). Nineteenth century Canada: Indigenous place of disease. *Health & Place, 4*(1), 55–66.

Human Potential Centre. (2015). *State of play survey: Executive report.* Auckland, New Zealand: Auckland University of Technology.

The Lawson Foundation. (2016). *Outdoor play strategy: An exploration of children's unstructured outdoor play in Canada.* Toronto: The Lawson Foundation.

Lester, S. (2013). Playing in a Deleuzian playground. In E. Ryall, W. Russell & M. MacLean (Eds.), *The philosophy of play*. Oxon, UK: Routledge.

Lester, S., & Russell, W. (2014). Turning the world upside down: Playing as the deliberate creation of uncertainty. *Children (Basel)*, *1*(2), 241–260.

Lupton, D. (1999). *Risk*. New York, NY: Routledge.

MacDonald, D., Abbott, R., Knez, K., & Nelson, A. (2009). Taking exercise: Cultural diversity and physically active lifestyles. *Sport, Education and Society*, *14*(1), 1–19.

MacDougall, C., Schiller, W., & Darbyshire, P. (2004). We have to live in the future. *Early Child Development and Care*, *174*(4), 369–387.

Norman, M. E., Petherick, L., Garcia, E., Glazebrook, C., Giesbrecht, G., & Todd Duhamel, T. (2015). Examining the more-than-built environments of a northern Manitoban community: Re-conceptualizing rural indigenous mobilities. *Journal of Rural Studies*, *42*, 166–178.

ParticipACTION. (2016). *Position statement on active outdoor play*. Ottawa, Canada: ParticipACTION.

PHAC. (2017). *Designing healthy living: The chief public health officer's report on the state of public health in Canada, 2017*. Ottawa, Canada: Public Health Agency of Canada. Retrieved December 2017 from www.canada.ca/en/public-health/services/publications/chief-public-health-officer-reports-state-public-health-canada/2017-designing-healthy-living.html

Postman, N. (1994). *The disappearance of childhood*. New York, NY: Vintage Books Inc.

Razack, S. (Ed.). (2002). *Race, space and the law: Unmapping a white settler society*. Toronto: Between the Lines Press.

Russell, W. (2013). Towards a spatial theory of playwork: What can Lefebvre offer as a response to playwork's inherent contradictions? In E. Ryall, W. Russell & M. MacLean (Eds.), *The philosophy of play* (pp. 164–174). London: Routledge.

Russell, W., Lester, S., Smith, H., MacLean, M., & Williams, T. (2016). *Sharing memories of adventure play (SMAP, 2016)*. Retrieved September 2017 from https://playandplaywork.com/2016/01/05/smap

Ryall, E., Russell, W., & Maclean, M. (2013). *The philosophy of play*. London: Routledge.

Sabo, D., & Veliz, P. (2008). *Go out and play: Youth sport in America*. East Meadow, NY: Women's Sport Foundation.

Sandseter, E. B. H. (2009). Characteristics of risky play. *Journal of Adventure Education and Outdoor Learning*, *9*(1), 3–21.

Sheerder, J., & Vandermeerschen, H. (2016). Playing an unequal game. Youth sport and social class. In K. Green & A. Smith (Eds.), *Routledge handbook of youth sport* (pp. 265–275). Oxon, UK: Routledge.

Silk, M., & Andrews, D. (2006). The fittest city in America. *Journal of Sport and Social Issues*, *30*(3), 315–327.

Sutton-Smith, B. (1997). *The ambiguity of play*. Boston, MA: Harvard University Press.

Taylor, T., & Doherty, A. (2005). Adolescent, sport, recreation and physical education: Experiences of recent arrivals to Canada. *Sport, Education and Society*, *10*(2), 211–238.

Tremblay, M. S., Barnes, J. D., Copeland, J., & Esliger, D. (2005). Conquering childhood inactivity: Is the answer in the past? *Medicine & Science in Sports & Exercise, 37*(7), 1187–1194.

Tremblay, M. S., Esliger, D., Copeland, J., Barnes, J., & Bassett, D. (2008). Moving forward by looking back: Lessons learned from long-lost lifestyles. *Applied Physiology, Nutrition, and Metabolism, 33*(4), 836–842.

Tremblay, M. S., Gray, C. E., Akinroye, K., Harrington, D. M., Katzmarzyk, P. T., Lambert, E. V., . . . Tomkinson, G. (2014). Physical activity of children: A global matrix of grades comparing 15 countries. *Journal of Physical Activity and Health, 11*(Suppl. 1), S113–S125. doi:10.1123/jpah.2014-0177

Truelove, S., Vanderloo, L. M., & Tucker, P. (2017). Defining and measuring active play among young children: A systematic review. *Journal of Physical Activity and Health, 14*, 155–166.

Vilhauer, M. (2013). Gadamer and the game of understanding: Dialogue-play and opening to others. In E. Ryall, W. Russell & M. MacLean (Eds.), *The philosophy of play* (pp. 75–86). London: Routledge.

Wall, J. (2013). All the world's a stage: Childhood and the play of being. In E. Ryall, W. Russell & M. MacLean (Eds.), *The philosophy of play* (pp. 32–43). London: Routledge.

Wexler, L., & Eglinton, K. (2015). Reconsidering youth well-being as fluid and relational: A dynamic process at the intersection of their physical and social geographies. In H. Cahill & J. Wyn (Eds.), *Handbook of children and youth studies* (pp. 127–137). New York, NY: Springer.

WHO. (2010). *Global recommendations on physical activity for health*. Geneva, Switzerland: World Health Organisation Press.

WHO. (2016). *Report of the commission on ending childhood obesity*. Geneva: World Health Organization Press.

Wortley, S., & Owusu-Bempah, A. (2014). The usual suspects: Police stop and search practices in Canada. *Policing and Society, 21*(4), 395–407.

Index

Note: Page numbers in *italics* indicate a figure.

Active Healthy Kids Canada: active play 53–55, 60–61, 62; development of active play concept 53–55, 57, 60–61, 62; play as pleasure 86, 87, 88–91; *Report Cards on Physical Activity* 3, 9, 50, 53–55, 85, 86, 113, 134–135, 142–144; risk in play 113–116, 120, 121; strategy for national prosperity 62–65, 69n1; *see also* Canadian Society for Exercise Physiology

active play: Active Healthy Kids Canada 53–55, 60–61, 62; Burrows, L. 68; Canadian Society for Exercise Physiology 50, 52, 57, 58; challenges in the promotion of 58–62; childhood obesity epidemic 48–52, 54, 58, 59, 60, 63; children's perspective on play 65–69; Chudacoff, H. 52; development of concept 53–58; exergames 57; fitness movement 61–62; Florence (study participant) 67; Foucault, M. 62; Freund, P. 51, 61; Henri (study participant) 68; instrumentalisation of 59–61; introduction 46, 46–48; Martin, G. 51, 61; measurement of 135–137; Michel (study participant) 66; ParticipACTION 53–55, 57, 60–61, 63–64, 69n1; public health considerations 46–62; *Push Play* 68; Russell, W. 61; screen time 51–52, 54–55, 58, 62; Sebastian (study participant) 65–66, 67–68; strategy for national prosperity 62–65; Sutton-Smith, B. 59

AHKC *see* Active Healthy Kids Canada
Alain (study participant) 93, 117

biopedagogy 11–12, 41–42, 63
biopolitics of risk 100, 101, 109, 117, 121; *see also* risk in play
biopower 11
Brown, S. 130–131
Bunton, R. 79–81
Burrows, L.: children's perspective on play 68; introduction 11, 12, 13; risk taking considerations 110, 113–114, 118

Caillois, R. 76–77, 130
Canadian Society for Exercise Physiology 50, 52, 57, 58; *see also* Active Healthy Kids Canada
Canadian Standards Association 105–106
Carla (study participant) 77
central argument, authors' 7–9; *see also* research methodology
chapter outlines 18–19
childhood obesity epidemic 48–52, 54, 58, 59, 60, 63
children's independent mobility 101–104, *103*
children's perspective on play: Alain (study participant) 93, 117; Arman (study participant) 106–107; Carla (study participant) 77; Eric (study participant) 92; Florence (study participant) 67; Henri (study participant) 68, 76; Marianne (study participant) 112; Michel (study

participant) 66, 110; Sarah (study participant) 92; Sebastian (study participant) 65–66, 67–68
child-saving movement 31, 33–34
Chudacoff, H.: active play 52; historical context of play 29–30, 32
CIM *see* children's independent mobility
Cohen, D. 38, 40
commodification of play 137–139
Coveney, J. 79–81
CSA *see* Canadian Standards Association
CSEP *see* Canadian Society for Exercise Physiology

definitions of different types of play 130–135; Brown, S. 130–131; Caillois, R. 130; *Position Statement on Active Outdoor Play* 134–135; "real play" 133–134; "risky play" 133; Ryall, E. 130; *see also* active play; free play
discourse analysis 16–17; *see also* theoretical approaches to play
Donnelly, P. 139–140

Eric (study participant) 92
ethics of pleasure 79–82; Bunton, R. 79–81; classical definition 79–80; Coveney, J. 79–81; Pronger, B. 81–82
eudaimonic pleasure 79
exergames 57

Florence (study participant) 67
Foucauldian theoretical concepts *see* Foucault, M.
Foucault, Michel: active play 62; biopower 11; institutional control of risk 109–110; playing as progress 41; theoretical approaches to play 9–11, 16
free play: historical context of play 37–38; introduction 2, 4, 6–7
free-range parenting 117–118
Freund, P. 51, 61
frivolous pleasure 85–91; differentiating child *versus* adult 85–86; Lupton, D. 90; promotion/modeling of play 87–91; Wellard, I. 88
Froebel, Friedrich 30–32
Frost, J. L. 27, 31–33

Global Alliance 142–144
Griffin, D. 118

Harwood, V. 11, 41–42
hedonic pleasure 79–82; Bunton, R. 79–81; classical definition 79–80; Coveney, J. 79–81; Pronger, B. 81–82
helicopter parenting 112, 132–133, 141
Henri (study participant) 68, 76
historical context of play: *The Ambiguity of Play* 39; biopedagogy 41–42; burgeoning public health discourse 40–43; child-saving movement 31, 33–34; Chudacoff, H. 29–30, 32; Cohen, D. 38, 40; contemporary perspectives 36–43; early evolution of play 28–36; evolving understanding of childhood development 28–30; free play 37–38; Froebel, F. 30–32; Frost, J. L. 27, 31–33; Huizinga, J. 5, 8; introduction 4–7, 26–27; kindergarten 31–34; Koch, Robert 31; Lester, S. 38; Nadesan, M. 41–42; "play as progress" 39–40; playground movement 31–36; play historians 4–5, 28–30; Reiger, K. M. 36; Russell, W. 38; Santer, J. 37; structured play 31–36; Sutton-Smith, B. 34, 37–38, 39
Homo Ludens 5, 36
Huizinga, J. 5, 8, 36

institutional control of risk 109–110; Foucault, M. 109–110; Michel (study participant) 110; *see also* risk in play
instrumentalisation: of active play 59–60; introduction 8; play, contemporary perspectives 40; play as pleasure 91
introduction: authors' central argument 7–9; authors' collaborative efforts 3–4; biopedagogy 11–12; biopower 11; Burrows, L. 11, 12, 13; chapter outlines 18–19; Foucault, M. 9–11, 16; free play 2, 4, 6–7; Harwood, V. 11; historical context of play 4–7, 10; *Homo Ludens* 5; Huizinga, J. 5, 8; instrumentalisation of play 8; neo-liberal influences in 12–14; photography notes 17–18; public health considerations 2–4, 7–10, 12–16, 18; research methodology

15–17; scope of book 1, 1–9; screen time 7, 15, 19; theoretical approaches to play 9–15

jouissance 79, 91

kindergarten 31–34; Froebel, F. 30–32
Koch, Robert 31
Kozlovksy, R. 42

Marianne (study participant) 112
Martin, G. 51, 61
McKendrick, J. 104
Michel (study participant) 66, 110

Nadesan, M. 41–42
necessity of outside play 113–119; Alain (study participant) 117; free-range parenting 117–118; Griffin, D. 118; Skenazy, L. 118; Tremblay, M. 114, 115
neo-liberal influences: in historical context of play 41; in play as pleasure 78, 83, 90; in public health considerations 12–14; in risk in play 110, 113; in theoretical approaches to play 12–14
nostalgic notions of play 139–142; Donnelly, P. 139–140; public health considerations 140–142

parental control of risk 110–113; Burrows, L. 111, 113–114; helicopter parenting phenomenon 112; Marianne (study participant) 112; risk regulation 110–113; see also risk in play
ParticipACTION: active play 53–55, 57, 60–61, 63–64, 69n1; development of active play concept 53–55, 57, 60–61; play as pleasure 86, 87, 88–91; risk in play 113–116, 120, 121; strategy for national prosperity 62–65, 69n1; see also Active Healthy Kids Canada
photography notes 17–18
play: active type 46, 46–69; The Ambiguity of Play 39; biopedagogy 41–42; burgeoning public health discourse 40–43; child-saving movement 31, 33–34; Chudacoff, H. 29–30, 32; Cohen, D. 38, 40; contemporary perspectives 36–43; definitions of different types of 130–135; early evolution of play 28–36; evolving understanding of childhood development 28–30; free play 2, 4, 6–7, 37–38, 53, 55, 102, 104, 109–110, 131, 140; Froebel, F. 30–32; Frost, J. L. 27, 31–33; Huizinga, J. 5, 8; introduction 4–7, 26–27; kindergarten 30–34; Koch, R. 31; Lester, S. 38; Nadesan, M. 41–42; necessity of outside type 113–119; nostalgic notions of 139–142; "play as progress" 39–40; playground considerations 31–36, 105–109; playground movement 31–36; play historians 4–5, 28–30; as pleasurable pastime 76, 76–94; Reiger, K. M. 36; risks associated with 98, 98–121, 103; Russell, W. 38; Santer, J. 37; as simple fun 129, 129–146; structured play 31–36; Sutton-Smith, B. 34, 37–38, 39; theoretical approaches to 9–16; see also children's perspective on play; public health considerations
play, children's perspective on: Alain (study participant) 93, 117; Arman (study participant) 106–107; Carla (study participant) 77; Eric (study participant) 92; Florence (study participant) 67; Henri (study participant) 68, 76; Marianne (study participant) 112; Michel (study participant) 66, 110; Sarah (study participant) 92; Sebastian (study participant) 65–66, 67–68
play, contemporary perspectives 36–43; The Ambiguity of Play 39; biopedagogy 41–42; burgeoning public health discourse 40–43; Cohen, D. 38; Foucault, M. 41; instrumentalisation of play 40; Kozlovksy, R. 42; Lester, S. 38; Nadesan, M. 41–42; "play as progress" 39–40; Russell, W. 38; Santer, J. 37; Sutton-Smith, B. 34, 37–38, 39
play as pleasure: Active Healthy Kids Canada 86, 87, 88–91; Alain (study participant) 93; Bunton, R. 79–81; Caillois, R. 76–77; Carla (study participant) 77; controlling pleasure 82–85; Coveney, J. 79–81; differentiating child versus adult types 85–86; Eric (study participant) 92; ethics of pleasure 79–82;

eudaimonic pleasure 79; frivolous pleasure 85–91; hedonic pleasure 79–82; instrumentalisation 91; introduction 76–79; jouissance 79, 91; neo-liberal influences in 78, 83, 90; ParticipACTION 86, 87, 88–91; pleasure control 82–85; pleasure types 77–98; promotion/modeling of play 87–91; Pronger, B. 81–82, 91; public health considerations 77–90, 94; Sarah (study participant) 92; summary of themes 91–94; Wellard, I. 88, 93–94; *see also* play as simple fun

"play as progress" 39–40

play as simple fun: Caillois, R. 130; commodification of play 137–139; definitions of different types of play 130–135; *Global Alliance* 142–144; *Global Matrix* 143; introduction 129, 129–130; measuring active play 135–137; nostalgic notions of 139–142; *Position Statement on Active Outdoor Play* 134–135; public health considerations 130–132, 137, 140, 141–142; "real play" 133–134; *Report Cards on Physical Activity* 142–144; "risky play" 133; Ryall, E. 130; summary of themes 144–146; World Health Organization 142–144; *see also* play as pleasure

playground considerations 31–36, 105–109; Arman (study participant) 106–107; Collyer, C. 106; playground movement 31–36; risk in play 105–109; *see also* historical context of play

playground movement 31–36; *see also* historical context of play

play historians 4–5, 28–30

pleasure control 82–85

pleasure types: Bunton, R. 79–81; Coveney, J. 79–81; ethics of pleasure 79–82; eudaimonic 79; hedonic 79–82; Pronger, B. 81–82, 91

Pronger, B. 81–82, 91

public health considerations: Active Healthy Kids Canada 53–55, 60–61, 63; active play 46, 46–62; author's collaborative efforts 3–4; authors' research methodology 15–17; biopedagogy 11, 41–42; biopower 11; burgeoning public health discourse 40–43; Burrows,

L. 68; Canadian Society for Exercise Physiology 50, 52, 57, 58; challenges in promoting active play 58–62; childhood obesity epidemic 48–52, 54, 58, 59, 60, 63; children's perspective on play 65–69; Chudacoff, H. 52; countering obesity epidemic 48–50; exergames 57; fitness movement 61–62; Foucault, M. 9–11, 16, 41, 62, 109–110; free play 2, 4, 6–7, 37–38; Freund, P. 51, 61; historical context of play 4–7, 10, 26, 26–43; *Homo Ludens* 5, 36; Huizinga, J. 5, 8, 36; Martin, G. 51, 61; Michel (study participant) 66; nostalgic notions of play 140–142; ParticipACTION 53–55, 57, 60–61, 63–64, 69n1; play as fun activity 77–90, 94; play as simple fun 130–132, 137, 140, 141–142; *Push Play* 68; risk in play 99, 101, 107, 109, 118–121; Russell, W. 61; screen time 51–52, 54–55, 58, 62; Sebastian (study participant) 65–66, 67–68; strategy for national prosperity 62–65; Sutton-Smith, B. 59; theoretical approaches to play 9–15

Push Play 68

Reiger, K. M. 36

Report Cards on Physical Activity 3, 9, 50, 53–55, 85, 86, 113, 134–135, 142–144; *see also* Active Healthy Kids Canada

research methodology 15–17; discourse analysis 16–17; objectives 15–16; *see also* central argument, authors'

risk in play: Alain (study participant) 117; Arman (study participant) 106–107; biopolitics of risk 100, 101, 109, 117, 121; Canadian Standards Association 105–106; children's independent mobility 101–104, *103*; Collyer, C. 106; free-range parenting 117–118; Griffin, D. 118; historical context 99–101; institutional control of risk 109–110; introduction *98*, 98–99; Marianne (study participant) 112; McKendrick, J. 104; necessity of outside play 113–119; neo-liberal influences in 111, 113; parental control of risk 110–113; ParticipACTION 113–116, 119, 120;

playground considerations 105–109; public health considerations 99, 101, 107, 109, 118–121; regulation of 109–113; Skenazy, L. 118; summary of themes 119–121; Tremblay, M. 114, 115; Valentine, G. 104

risk regulation: institutional control 109–110; parental control 110–113

Russell, W. 61

Ryall, E. 130

Sarah (study participant) 92

scope of book *1*, 1–9

screen time: active play 51–52, 54–55, 58, 62; introduction 7, 15, 19

Sebastian (study participant) 65–66, 67–68

Skenazy, L. 118

strategy for national prosperity: Active Healthy Kids Canada 63–64, 69n1; active play 62–65; ParticipACTION 63–64, 69n1

Sutton-Smith, B.: active play 59; historical context of play 34, 37–38, 39; "play as progress" 39–40

theoretical approaches to play 9–16; biopedagogy 11–12; biopower 11; Burrows, L. 11, 12, 13; Foucault, M. 9–11, 16; Harwood, V. 11; neo-liberal influences in 12–14

Tremblay, M. 114, 115

Twain, M. 26

Valentine, G. 104

Wellard, I. 88, 93–94

WHO *see* World Health Organization

World Health Organization 48–49, 142–144